Student Worksheets

Visual Anatomy & Physiology

Second Edition

Frederic H. Martini, Ph.D.
University of Hawaii at Manoa

William C. Ober, M.D.
Washington and Lee University

Judi L. Nath, Ph.D.
Lourdes University, Sylvania, Ohio

Edwin F. Bartholomew, M.S.

Kevin Petti, Ph.D.
San Diego Miramar College

Claire E. Ober, R.N.
Illustrator

Kathleen Welch, M.D.
Clinical Consultant

Ralph T. Hutchings
Biomedical Photographer

PEARSON

Boston   Columbus   Indianapolis   New York   San Francisco   Upper Saddle River
Amsterdam   Cape Town   Dubai   London   Madrid   Milan   Munich   Paris   Montréal   Toronto
Delhi   Mexico City   São Paulo   Sydney   Hong Kong   Seoul   Singapore   Taipei   Tokyo

Executive Editor: *Leslie Berriman*
Associate Project Editor: *Lisa Damerel*
Assistant Editor: *Cady Owens*
Editorial Assistant: *Sharon Kim*
Director of Development: *Barbara Yien*
Development Editor: *Molly Ward*
Managing Editor: *Mike Early*
Assistant Managing Editor: *Nancy Tabor*
Production Management and Composition: *S4Carlisle Publishing Services, Inc.*
Design Manager: *Mark Ong*
Interior Designer: *Gibson Design Associates*

Main Text Cover Designer: *tani hasegawa*
Supplement Cover Designer: *Seventeenth Street Studios*
Art House: *Precision Graphics*
Contributing Illustrators: *imagineeringart.com; Anita Impagliazzo*
Photo Permissions Management: *Bill Smith Group*
Photo Researchers: *Stefanie Ramsay; Luke Malone; Cordes Hoffman*
Associate Director of Image Management: *Travis Amos*
Senior Procurement Specialist: *Stacey Weinberger*
Senior Anatomy & Physiology Specialist: *Derek Perrigo*
Senior Marketing Manager: *Allison Rona*

Cover Photo Credit: © Alexander Yakovlev/Shutterstock

Credits and acknowledgments for materials borrowed from other sources and reproduced, with permission, in this textbook appear after the Answers.

Notice: Our knowledge in clinical sciences is constantly changing. The authors and the publisher of this volume have taken care that the information contained herein is accurate and compatible with the standards generally accepted at the time of the publication. Nevertheless, it is difficult to ensure that all information given is entirely accurate for all circumstances. The authors and the publisher disclaim any liability, loss, or damage incurred as a consequence, directly or indirectly, of the use and application of any of the contents of this volume.

ISBN 10: **0-321-95631-1**; ISBN 13: **978-0-321-95631-6** (Stand-alone)
ISBN 10: **0-321-98073-5**; ISBN 13: **978-0-321-98073-1** (ValuePack)

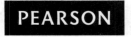

Contents

Visual Anatomy & Physiology, Second Edition is designed with frequent opportunities to pause and practice, helping you to pace your learning throughout each chapter. This workbook gives you a space outside of your book to complete the Section Reviews and Chapter Review Questions.

Each of the **Section Review** pages from the textbook is reproduced twice in this workbook, so you can work through these exercises more than once—without writing in your textbook. Complete each Section Review once while reading the chapter and again right before your exam to help you review the material. Answers to the Section Reviews are included at the back of this workbook.

The **Chapter Review Questions** from the end of each chapter in your textbook are also included in this workbook. Each question is reproduced with space for you to write. The answers to the Chapter Review Questions are included at the back of this workbook.

Don't forget: Lots of additional practice is available in the Study Area of **MasteringA&P**®. Practice Anatomy Lab™ (PAL™), A&P Flix™ animations, MP3 Tutor Sessions, Interactive Physiology®, and PhysioEx™ are all included to help you succeed in your A&P course.

Vocabulary

For each of the following descriptions, write the appropriate characteristic of living things in the corresponding blank.

1 Usually refers to the absorption and utilization of oxygen and the generation and release of carbon dioxide

2 Produces organisms characteristic of its species

3 Changes in the behavior, capabilities, or structure of an organism

4 Movement of fluid within the body; may involve a pump and a network of special vessels

5 Elimination of chemical waste products generated by the body

6 Chemical breakdown of complex structures for absorption and use by the body

7 Transports materials around the body of a large organism; changes orientation or position of a plant or immobile animal; moves mobile animals around the environment (locomotion)

8 Indicates that the organism recognizes changes in the internal or external environment

1 _____

2 _____

3 _____

4 _____

5 _____

6 _____

7 _____

8 _____

Write each of the following terms under the proper heading.

- Right atrium
- Myocardium
- Valve to aorta opens
- Left ventricle
- Valve between left atrium and left ventricle closes
- Pressure in left atrium
- Electrocardiogram
- Endocardium
- Superior vena cava
- Heartbeat

9 Anatomy

_____

_____

_____

_____

_____

10 Physiology

_____

_____

_____

_____

_____

Short answer

Briefly describe how the relationship of form and function of a house key and its front door lock are both similar to and different from a chemical messenger and its receptor molecule.

11 _____

_____

_____

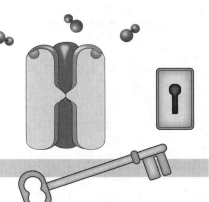

Section integration

How might a large organism's survival be affected by an inadequate internal circulation network?

12 _____

_____

Vocabulary

For each of the following descriptions, write the appropriate characteristic of living things in the corresponding blank.

1 Usually refers to the absorption and utilization of oxygen and the generation and release of carbon dioxide

2 Produces organisms characteristic of its species

3 Changes in the behavior, capabilities, or structure of an organism

4 Movement of fluid within the body; may involve a pump and a network of special vessels

5 Elimination of chemical waste products generated by the body

6 Chemical breakdown of complex structures for absorption and use by the body

7 Transports materials around the body of a large organism; changes orientation or position of a plant or immobile animal; moves mobile animals around the environment (locomotion)

8 Indicates that the organism recognizes changes in the internal or external environment

1 _____

2 _____

3 _____

4 _____

5 _____

6 _____

7 _____

8 _____

Write each of the following terms under the proper heading.

- Right atrium
- Myocardium
- Valve to aorta opens
- Left ventricle
- Valve between left atrium and left ventricle closes
- Pressure in left atrium
- Electrocardiogram
- Endocardium
- Superior vena cava
- Heartbeat

9 Anatomy

_____

_____

_____

_____

_____

10 Physiology

_____

_____

_____

_____

_____

Short answer

Briefly describe how the relationship of form and function of a house key and its front door lock are both similar to and different from a chemical messenger and its receptor molecule.

11 _____

_____

_____

Section integration

How might a large organism's survival be affected by an inadequate internal circulation network?

12 _____

_____

Concept map

Use each of the following terms once to fill in the blank boxes to correctly complete the map.

- organs
- epithelial tissue
- cells
- connective tissue
- muscle tissue
- neural tissue
- organ systems
- external and internal surfaces
- matrix
- glandular secretions
- bones of the skeleton
- neuroglia
- blood
- materials within digestive tract
- protein fibers
- ground substance
- movement

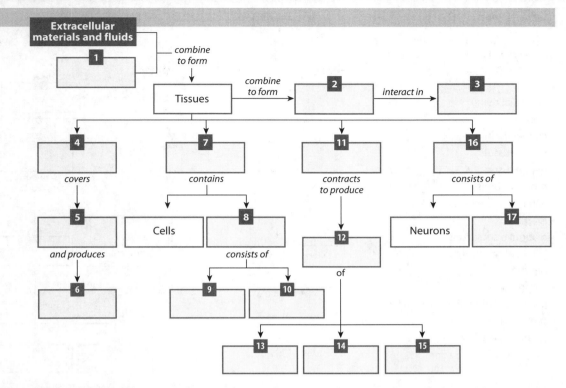

Vocabulary

Reorder the levels of organization listed below into the correct sequence from simplest to most complex.

- organ system
- organ
- tissue
- chemical
- organism
- cellular

18 _____
_____
_____

Short answer

Summarize the major functions of each of the following organ systems.

19 Integumentary   19 _____
20 Skeletal   20 _____
21 Muscular   21 _____
22 Nervous   22 _____
23 Endocrine   23 _____
24 Cardiovascular   24 _____

25 Lymphatic   25 _____
26 Respiratory   26 _____
27 Digestive   27 _____
28 Urinary   28 _____
29 Reproductive   29 _____

Section integration

For five different organ systems in the human body, identify a specialized cell type found in that system.

30 _____
_____
_____
_____

Concept map

Use each of the following terms once to fill in the blank boxes to correctly complete the map.

- organs
- epithelial tissue
- cells
- connective tissue
- muscle tissue
- neural tissue
- organ systems
- external and internal surfaces
- matrix
- glandular secretions
- bones of the skeleton
- neuroglia
- blood
- materials within digestive tract
- protein fibers
- ground substance
- movement

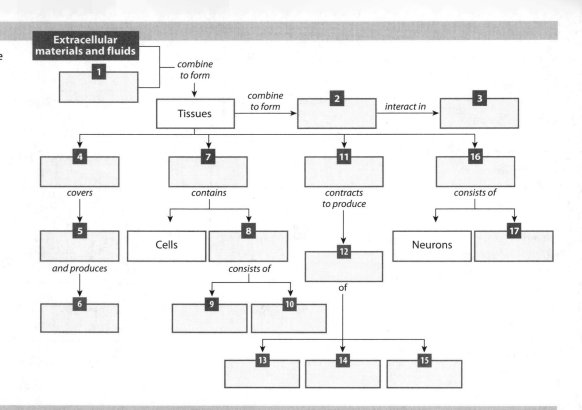

Vocabulary

Reorder the levels of organization listed below into the correct sequence from simplest to most complex.

- organ system
- tissue
- organism
- organ
- chemical
- cellular

18 _____
_____
_____

Short answer

Summarize the major functions of each of the following organ systems.

19	Integumentary	19 _____
20	Skeletal	20 _____
21	Muscular	21 _____
22	Nervous	22 _____
23	Endocrine	23 _____
24	Cardiovascular	24 _____

25	Lymphatic	25 _____
26	Respiratory	26 _____
27	Digestive	27 _____
28	Urinary	28 _____
29	Reproductive	29 _____

Section integration

For five different organ systems in the human body, identify a specialized cell type found in that system.

30 _____
_____
_____
_____

Vocabulary

Write the term for each of the following descriptions in the space provided.

1 Mechanism that increases a deviation from normal limits after an initial stimulus

2 Adjustment of physiological systems to preserve homeostasis

3 The maintenance of a relatively constant internal environment

4 Homeostatic regulatory component that detects changes

5 Corrective mechanism that opposes or cancels a variation from normal limits

1 _____

2 _____

3 _____

4 _____

5 _____

Indicate whether each of the following processes represents negative feedback or positive feedback.

6 A rise in the level of calcium dissolved in the blood stimulates the release of a hormone that causes bone cells to deposit more of the calcium in bone.

7 Labor contractions become increasingly forceful during childbirth.

8 An increase in blood pressure triggers a nervous system response that results in lowering the blood pressure.

9 Blood vessel cells damaged by a break in the vessel release chemicals that accelerate the blood clotting process.

6 _____

7 _____

8 _____

9 _____

Short answer

Assuming a normal body temperature range of 36.7°–37.2°C (98°–99°F), identify from the graph below what would happen if there were an increase or decrease in body temperature beyond the normal limits. Use the following descriptive terms to explain what would happen at (10) and (11) on the graph.

- body surface cools
- shivering occurs
- sweating increases
- temperature declines
- body heat is conserved
- blood flow to skin increases
- blood flow to skin decreases
- temperature rises

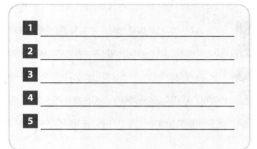

37.8°C/100°F

36.7°–37.2°C/98°–99°F

36.1°C/97°F

10

11

] Normal range

10 _____
_____
_____
_____

11 _____
_____
_____
_____

Section integration

It is a warm day and you feel a little chilled. On checking your temperature, you find that your body temperature is 1.5 degrees below normal. Suggest some possible reasons for this situation.

12 _____
_____
_____
_____

Vocabulary

Write the term for each of the following descriptions in the space provided.

1 Mechanism that increases a deviation from normal limits after an initial stimulus

2 Adjustment of physiological systems to preserve homeostasis

3 The maintenance of a relatively constant internal environment

4 Homeostatic regulatory component that detects changes

5 Corrective mechanism that opposes or cancels a variation from normal limits

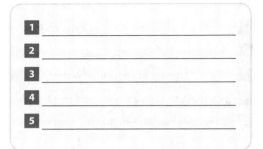

Indicate whether each of the following processes represents negative feedback or positive feedback.

6 A rise in the level of calcium dissolved in the blood stimulates the release of a hormone that causes bone cells to deposit more of the calcium in bone.

7 Labor contractions become increasingly forceful during childbirth.

8 An increase in blood pressure triggers a nervous system response that results in lowering the blood pressure.

9 Blood vessel cells damaged by a break in the vessel release chemicals that accelerate the blood clotting process.

Short answer

Assuming a normal body temperature range of 36.7°–37.2°C (98°–99°F), identify from the graph below what would happen if there were an increase or decrease in body temperature beyond the normal limits. Use the following descriptive terms to explain what would happen at (10) and (11) on the graph.

- body surface cools
- shivering occurs
- sweating increases
- temperature declines
- body heat is conserved
- blood flow to skin increases
- blood flow to skin decreases
- temperature rises

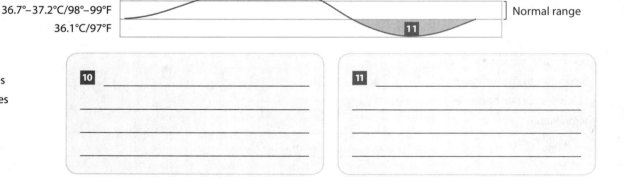

10

11

Section integration

It is a warm day and you feel a little chilled. On checking your temperature, you find that your body temperature is 1.5 degrees below normal. Suggest some possible reasons for this situation.

12

Labeling

Label the directional terms in the figures at right.

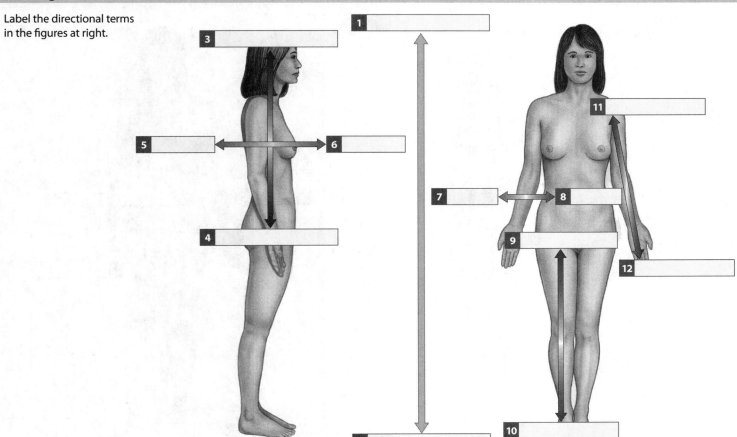

Concept map

Use each of the following terms once to fill in the blank boxes to correctly complete the body cavities concept map.

- digestive glands and organs
- abdominopelvic cavity
- thoracic cavity
- heart
- mediastinum
- diaphragm
- pelvic cavity
- trachea, esophagus
- reproductive organs
- left lung
- peritoneal cavity

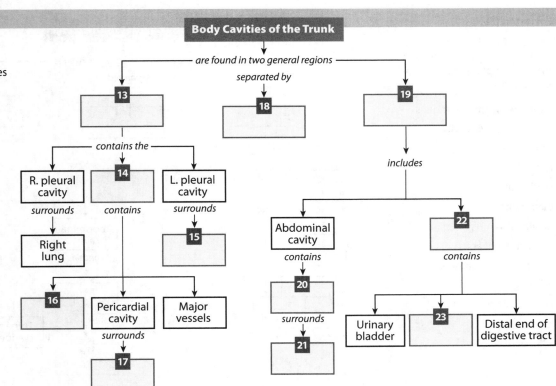

Labeling

Label the directional terms in the figures at right.

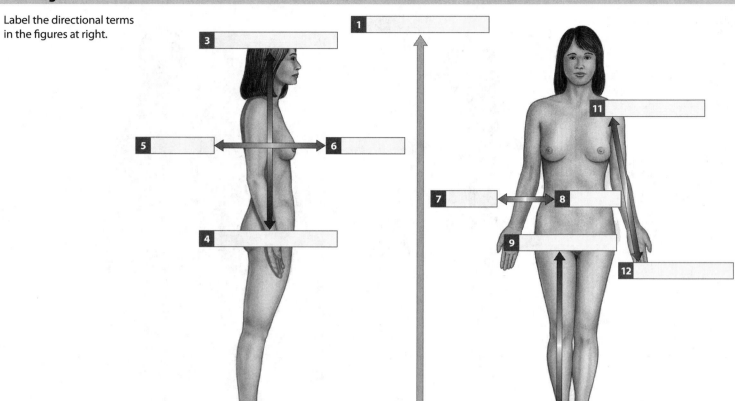

Concept map

Use each of the following terms once to fill in the blank boxes to correctly complete the body cavities concept map.

- digestive glands and organs
- abdominopelvic cavity
- thoracic cavity
- heart
- mediastinum
- diaphragm
- pelvic cavity
- trachea, esophagus
- reproductive organs
- left lung
- peritoneal cavity

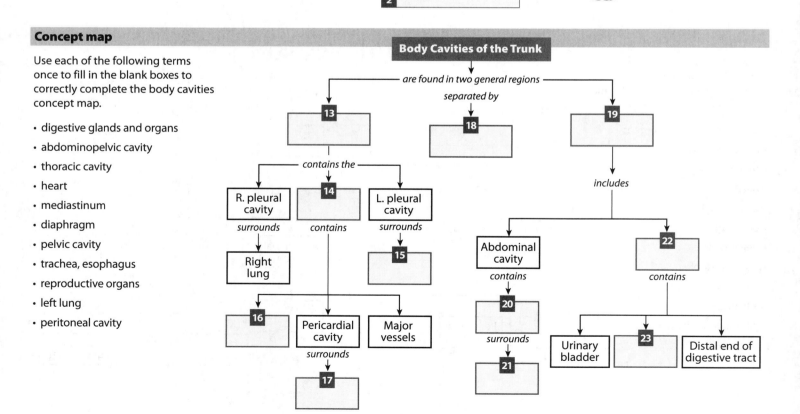

Chapter Review Questions

Labeling

Identify the body cavities as well as the organs they enclose.

1 _____

2 _____

3 _____

4 _____

5 _____

6 _____

Matching

Match each lettered term with the most closely related description.

a. cytology
b. physiology
c. histology
d. anatomy
e. homeostasis
f. muscle
g. heart
h. endocrine
i. temperature regulation
j. labor and delivery
k. supine
l. prone
m. abdominopelvic cavity
n. pericardium

7 _____ Study of tissues

8 _____ Constant internal environment

9 _____ Face up position

10 _____ Study of functions

11 _____ Positive feedback

12 _____ Organ system

13 _____ Study of cells

14 _____ Negative feedback

15 _____ Serous membrane

16 _____ Study of internal and external body structures

17 _____ Diaphragm tissue

18 _____ Peritoneal cavity

19 _____ Organ

20 _____ Face down position

Multiple choice

Select the correct answer from the list provided.

21 What is the correct order, from simplest to most complex, of the six levels of organization that make up the human body?

- [ ] a) cell, chemical, tissue, organ, organ system, organism
- [ ] b) chemical, cell, tissue, organ, organ system, organism
- [ ] c) chemical, cell, tissue, organ system, organ, organism
- [ ] d) chemical, cell, organ, tissue, organ system, organism
- [ ] e) cell, tissue, chemical, organ, organism, organ system

22 The increasingly forceful labor contractions during childbirth are an example of

- [ ] a) receptor activation.
- [ ] b) effector shutdown.
- [ ] c) negative feedback.
- [ ] d) positive feedback.

23 A plane through the body that passes perpendicular to the long axis of the body and divides the body into a superior and an inferior section is a

☐ a) sagittal section.

☐ b) transverse section.

☐ c) coronal section.

☐ d) frontal section.

24 The mediastinum is the region between the

☐ a) lungs and heart.

☐ b) two pleural cavities.

☐ c) chest and abdomen.

☐ d) heart and pericardium.

25 The unit used to measure cell dimensions is the

☐ a) centimeter (cm).

☐ b) millimeter (mm).

☐ c) micrometer (μm).

☐ d) kilometer (km).

26 The two major body cavities of the trunk are the

☐ a) pleural cavity and pericardial cavity.

☐ b) pericardial cavity and peritoneal cavity.

☐ c) pleural cavity and peritoneal cavity.

☐ d) thoracic cavity and abdominopelvic cavity.

27 Which of the following is *not* a characteristic of life?

☐ a) responsiveness

☐ b) movement

☐ c) manipulation of external environment

☐ d) reproduction

28 Which sectional plane would divide the body so that the face remains intact?

☐ a) sagittal plane

☐ b) frontal (coronal) plane

☐ c) midsagittal plane

☐ d) parasagittal plane

Short answer

29 Define anatomy. Define physiology.

_____

_____

_____

30 Describe the three basic principles of the cell theory.

_____

_____

_____

31 In which body cavity would each of the following organs be enclosed? Heart, small intestine, large intestine, lung, kidneys.

_____

_____

_____

32 Identify each of the four primary tissue types and give an example of where in the body that tissue would be found.

_____

_____

_____

33 The hormone calcitonin is released from the thyroid gland in response to increased levels of calcium ions in the blood. If this hormone is controlled by negative feedback, what effect would calcitonin have on blood calcium levels?

_____

_____

_____

34 A stroke occurs when there is a disruption in blood flow to the brain, causing brain cells to die. Predict the kind of symptoms a stroke patient would have. Apply your knowledge of organ system function.

_____

_____

_____

Matching

Match each lettered term with the most closely related description.

a. atomic number

b. electrons

c. protons

d. neutrons

e. isotopes

f. ions

g. ionic bond

h. covalent bond

i. mass number

j. element

k. compound

l. hydrogen bond

1	Atoms that have gained or lost electrons
2	Subatomic particles in the nucleus, have no electrical charge
3	Atoms of two or more different elements bonded together in a fixed proportion
4	The number of protons in an atom
5	Attractive force between water molecules
6	Type of chemical bond within a water molecule
7	The number of subatomic particles in the nucleus
8	Substance composed only of atoms with same atomic number
9	Subatomic particles in the nucleus, have an electrical charge
10	Atoms of the same element with different masses
11	Type of chemical bond in table salt
12	Subatomic particles outside the nucleus, have an electrical charge

1 _____
2 _____
3 _____
4 _____
5 _____
6 _____
7 _____
8 _____
9 _____
10 _____
11 _____
12 _____

Fill-in

Fill in the missing information in the following table.

Element	Number of protons	Number of electrons	Number of neutrons	Mass number
Helium	13	2	2	14
Hydrogen	1	15	16	1
Carbon	6	17	6	18
Nitrogen	19	7	20	14
Calcium	21	22	20	40

Indicate which of the following molecules are also compounds.

 H_2 (hydrogen) H_2O (water) O_2 (oxygen)   CO (carbon monoxide)

23 _____   24 _____   25 _____   26 _____

Section integration

Describe how the following pairs of terms concerning atomic interactions are similar and how they are different.

27 Inert element/reactive element

28 Polar molecules/nonpolar molecules

29 Covalent bond/ionic bond

27 _____
_____

28 _____
_____

29 _____
_____

Matching

Match each lettered term with the most closely related description.

a. atomic number

b. electrons

c. protons

d. neutrons

e. isotopes

f. ions

g. ionic bond

h. covalent bond

i. mass number

j. element

k. compound

l. hydrogen bond

1 Atoms that have gained or lost electrons

2 Subatomic particles in the nucleus, have no electrical charge

3 Atoms of two or more different elements bonded together in a fixed proportion

4 The number of protons in an atom

5 Attractive force between water molecules

6 Type of chemical bond within a water molecule

7 The number of subatomic particles in the nucleus

8 Substance composed only of atoms with same atomic number

9 Subatomic particles in the nucleus, have an electrical charge

10 Atoms of the same element with different masses

11 Type of chemical bond in table salt

12 Subatomic particles outside the nucleus, have an electrical charge

1 _____

2 _____

3 _____

4 _____

5 _____

6 _____

7 _____

8 _____

9 _____

10 _____

11 _____

12 _____

Fill-in

Fill in the missing information in the following table.

Element	Number of protons	Number of electrons	Number of neutrons	Mass number
Helium	**13**	2	2	**14**
Hydrogen	1	**15**	**16**	1
Carbon	6	**17**	6	**18**
Nitrogen	**19**	7	**20**	14
Calcium	**21**	**22**	20	40

Indicate which of the following molecules are also compounds.

H_2 (hydrogen)

H_2O (water)

O_2 (oxygen)

CO (carbon monoxide)

23 [_____]

24 [_____]

25 [_____]

26 [_____]

Section integration

Describe how the following pairs of terms concerning atomic interactions are similar and how they are different.

27 Inert element/reactive element

28 Polar molecules/nonpolar molecules

29 Covalent bond/ionic bond

27 _____
_____

28 _____
_____

29 _____
_____

Matching

Match each lettered term with the most closely related description.

a. exergonic

b. activation energy

c. organic compounds

d. exchange reaction

e. hydrolysis

f. endergonic

g. reactants

h. enzyme

1 Catalyst

2 Starting substances in a chemical reaction

3 Chemical reaction involving water

4 Reactions that absorb energy

5 Shuffles parts of reactants

6 Primary components are carbon and hydrogen

7 Reactions that release energy

8 Requirement for starting a chemical reaction

1 _____

2 _____

3 _____

4 _____

5 _____

6 _____

7 _____

8 _____

Short answer

Using chemical notation, write the formula of each of the following:

9 One molecule of hydrogen

10 Two atoms of hydrogen

11 Six molecules of water

12 One molecule of sucrose (in this order: 12 atoms of carbon, 22 atoms of hydrogen, and 11 atoms of oxygen)

9 _____

10 _____

11 _____

12 _____

Write the chemical equation for the following chemical reaction: one molecule of glucose combined with six molecules of oxygen produce six molecules of carbon dioxide and six molecules of water.

13 _____

Indicate which of the following is a hydrolysis reaction and which is a dehydration synthesis reaction.

14 $A\text{—}B + H_2O \longrightarrow A\text{—}H + HO\text{—}B$

15 $A\text{—}H + HO\text{—}B \longrightarrow A\text{—}B + H_2O$

14 _____

15 _____

Section integration

In a metabolic pathway that consists of four steps, how would decreasing the amount of enzyme that catalyzes the second step affect the amount of product at the end of the pathway?

16 _____

_____

Matching

Match each lettered term with the most closely related description.

a. exergonic

b. activation energy

c. organic compounds

d. exchange reaction

e. hydrolysis

f. endergonic

g. reactants

h. enzyme

1 Catalyst

2 Starting substances in a chemical reaction

3 Chemical reaction involving water

4 Reactions that absorb energy

5 Shuffles parts of reactants

6 Primary components are carbon and hydrogen

7 Reactions that release energy

8 Requirement for starting a chemical reaction

1 _____

2 _____

3 _____

4 _____

5 _____

6 _____

7 _____

8 _____

Short answer

Using chemical notation, write the formula of each of the following:

9 One molecule of hydrogen

10 Two atoms of hydrogen

11 Six molecules of water

12 One molecule of sucrose (in this order: 12 atoms of carbon, 22 atoms of hydrogen, and 11 atoms of oxygen)

9 _____

10 _____

11 _____

12 _____

Write the chemical equation for the following chemical reaction: one molecule of glucose combined with six molecules of oxygen produce six molecules of carbon dioxide and six molecules of water.

13 _____

Indicate which of the following is a hydrolysis reaction and which is a dehydration synthesis reaction.

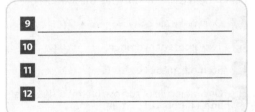

14 $A\text{—}B + H_2O \longrightarrow A\text{—}H + HO\text{—}B$

15 $A\text{—}H + HO\text{—}B \longrightarrow A\text{—}B + H_2O$

14 _____

15 _____

Section integration

In a metabolic pathway that consists of four steps, how would decreasing the amount of enzyme that catalyzes the second step affect the amount of product at the end of the pathway?

16 _____

_____

Matching

Match each lettered term with the most closely related description.

a. solvent

b. water

c. buffers

d. hydrophilic

e. inorganic compounds

f. hydrophobic

g. acid

h. solute

i. alkaline

j. salt

1 HCl, NaOH, and NaCl

2 A dissolved substance

3 A solution with a pH greater than 7

4 Molecules that readily interact with water

5 Fluid medium of a solution

6 Ionic compound not containing hydrogen ions or hydroxide ions

7 Compounds that stabilize pH in body fluids

8 Solution with a pH of 6.5

9 Molecules that do not interact with water

10 Makes up two-thirds of human body weight

1 _____

2 _____

3 _____

4 _____

5 _____

6 _____

7 _____

8 _____

9 _____

10 _____

Short answer

List four properties of water important to the functioning of the human body.

11 _____

12 _____

13 _____

14 _____

Identify the regions 15, 16, and 17 on the pH scale below:

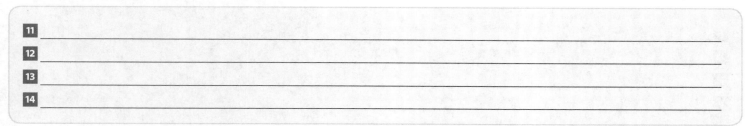

pH	0	1	2	3	4	5	6	7	8	9	10	11	12	13	14
$[H^+]$ (mol/L)	10^0	10^{-1}	10^{-2}	10^{-3}	10^{-4}	10^{-5}	10^{-6}	10^{-7}	10^{-8}	10^{-9}	10^{-10}	10^{-11}	10^{-12}	10^{-13}	10^{-14}

18 How much more or less acidic is a solution of pH 3 compared to one with a pH of 6?

18 _____

19 Describe three negative effects of abnormal pH fluctuations in the human body.

19 _____

Section integration

The addition of table salt to pure water does not result in a change in its pH. Why?

20 _____

Matching

Match each lettered term with the most closely related description.

a. solvent

b. water

c. buffers

d. hydrophilic

e. inorganic compounds

f. hydrophobic

g. acid

h. solute

i. alkaline

j. salt

1 HCl, NaOH, and NaCl

2 A dissolved substance

3 A solution with a pH greater than 7

4 Molecules that readily interact with water

5 Fluid medium of a solution

6 Ionic compound not containing hydrogen ions or hydroxide ions

7 Compounds that stabilize pH in body fluids

8 Solution with a pH of 6.5

9 Molecules that do not interact with water

10 Makes up two-thirds of human body weight

1 _____

2 _____

3 _____

4 _____

5 _____

6 _____

7 _____

8 _____

9 _____

10 _____

Short answer

List four properties of water important to the functioning of the human body.

11 _____

12 _____

13 _____

14 _____

Identify the regions 15, 16, and 17 on the pH scale below:

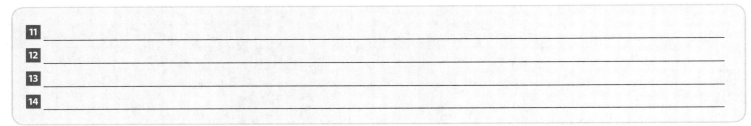

| 16 |
| 15 |
| 17 |

pH	0	1	2	3	4	5	6	7	8	9	10	11	12	13	14
[H⁺] (mol/L)	10^0	10^{-1}	10^{-2}	10^{-3}	10^{-4}	10^{-5}	10^{-6}	10^{-7}	10^{-8}	10^{-9}	10^{-10}	10^{-11}	10^{-12}	10^{-13}	10^{-14}

18 How much more or less acidic is a solution of pH 3 compared to one with a pH of 6?

18 _____

19 Describe three negative effects of abnormal pH fluctuations in the human body.

19 _____

Section integration

The addition of table salt to pure water does not result in a change in its pH. Why?

20 _____

Concept map

Use each of the following terms once to fill in the blank boxes to correctly complete the organic compounds concept map.

- lipids
- carbohydrates
- nucleic acids
- disaccharides
- RNA
- fatty acids
- phosphate groups
- glycerol
- polysaccharides
- proteins
- monosaccharides
- ATP
- amino acids
- DNA
- nucleotides

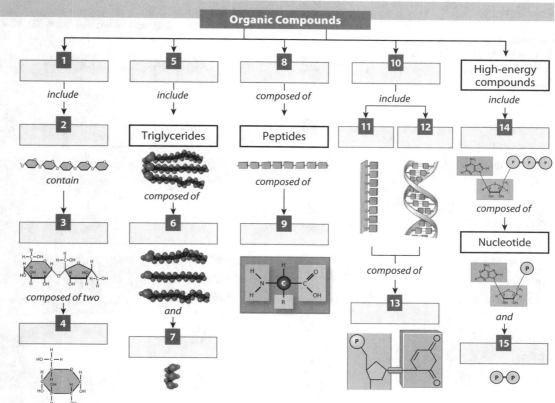

Vocabulary

In the space provided, write the boldfaced terms introduced in this section that contain the indicated word part.

| 16 | poly- *(many)* | 16 _____ |
| 17 | tri- *(three)* | 17 _____ |

| 18 | di- *(two)* | 18 _____ |
| 19 | glyco- *(sugar)* | 19 _____ |

Matching

Match each lettered term with the most closely related description.

a. monosaccharide
b. ATP
c. polyunsaturated
d. glycerol
e. cholesterol
f. isomers
g. glycogen
h. active site
i. nucleotide
j. RNA
k. peptide

20 Polysaccharide with an energy-storage role in animal tissues

21 Molecules with same chemical formula but different structure

22 A fatty acid with more than one C-to-C double covalent bond

23 The region of an enzyme that binds the substrate

24 Three-carbon molecule that combines with fatty acids

25 A steroid essential to plasma membranes

26 A high-energy compound consisting of adenosine and three phosphate groups

27 A nucleic acid that contains the sugar ribose

28 The covalent bond between the carboxylic acid and amino groups of adjacent amino acids

29 Organic molecule consisting of a sugar, a phosphate group, and a nitrogenous base

30 A simple sugar

20 _____
21 _____
22 _____
23 _____
24 _____
25 _____
26 _____
27 _____
28 _____
29 _____
30 _____

Concept map

Use each of the following terms once to fill in the blank boxes to correctly complete the organic compounds concept map.

- lipids
- carbohydrates
- nucleic acids
- disaccharides
- RNA
- fatty acids
- phosphate groups
- glycerol
- polysaccharides
- proteins
- monosaccharides
- ATP
- amino acids
- DNA
- nucleotides

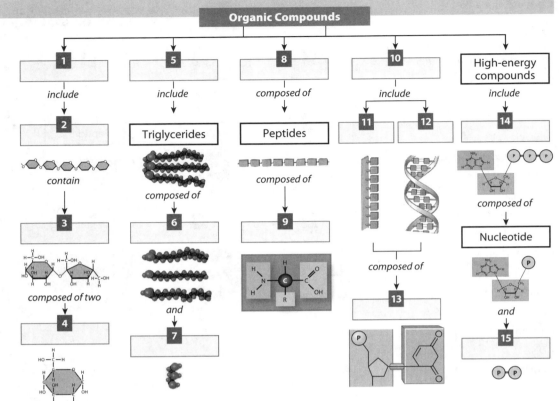

Organic Compounds

| 1 | 5 | 8 | 10 | High-energy compounds |

include — include — composed of — include — include

| 2 | Triglycerides | Peptides | 11 | 12 | 14 |

contain — composed of — composed of

| 3 | 6 | 9 | composed of | Nucleotide |

composed of two — composed of — composed of

| 4 | 7 | 13 | and | 15 |

and

Vocabulary

In the space provided, write the boldfaced terms introduced in this section that contain the indicated word part.

16 poly- *(many)* 16 _____

17 tri- *(three)* 17 _____

18 di- *(two)* 18 _____

19 glyco- *(sugar)* 19 _____

Matching

Match each lettered term with the most closely related description.

a. monosaccharide

b. ATP

c. polyunsaturated

d. glycerol

e. cholesterol

f. isomers

g. glycogen

h. active site

i. nucleotide

j. RNA

k. peptide

20 Polysaccharide with an energy-storage role in animal tissues   20 _____

21 Molecules with same chemical formula but different structure   21 _____

22 A fatty acid with more than one C-to-C double covalent bond   22 _____

23 The region of an enzyme that binds the substrate   23 _____

24 Three-carbon molecule that combines with fatty acids   24 _____

25 A steroid essential to plasma membranes   25 _____

26 A high-energy compound consisting of adenosine and three phosphate groups   26 _____

27 A nucleic acid that contains the sugar ribose   27 _____

28 The covalent bond between the carboxylic acid and amino groups of adjacent amino acids   28 _____

29 Organic molecule consisting of a sugar, a phosphate group, and a nitrogenous base   29 _____

30 A simple sugar   30 _____

Chapter Review Questions

Multiple choice

Select the correct answer from the list provided.

1 If a polypeptide contains 10 peptide bonds, how many amino acids does it contain?
- ☐ a) 9
- ☐ b) 10
- ☐ c) 11
- ☐ d) 12

2 A dehydration synthesis reaction between glycerol and a single fatty acid would yield a(n)
- ☐ a) micelle.
- ☐ b) omega-3 fatty acid.
- ☐ c) monoglyceride.
- ☐ d) diglyceride.

3 An atom of calcium has 20 protons and 20 neutrons. What is its atomic number?
- ☐ a) 10
- ☐ b) 20
- ☐ c) 40
- ☐ d) 60

4 In an exergonic reaction,
- ☐ a) large molecules are broken down into smaller ones.
- ☐ b) small molecules are assembled into larger ones.
- ☐ c) molecules are rearranged to form new molecules.
- ☐ d) molecules move from reactants to products and back.
- ☐ e) energy is released during the reaction.

5 The hydrogen bonding that occurs in water is responsible for all of the following, except
- ☐ a) the high boiling point of water.
- ☐ b) the low freezing point of water.
- ☐ c) the ability of water to dissolve nonpolar substances.
- ☐ d) the ability of water to dissolve inorganic salts.
- ☐ e) the high surface tension of water.

6 The subatomic particle with the least mass
- ☐ a) carries a negative charge.
- ☐ b) carries a positive charge.
- ☐ c) plays no part in the atom's chemical reactions.
- ☐ d) is found only in the nucleus.

7 A(n) _____ forms when atoms interact to produce larger, more complex structures.
- ☐ a) isotope
- ☐ b) enzyme
- ☐ c) molecule
- ☐ d) nucleus

8 Isotopes of an element differ from each other in the number of
- ☐ a) protons in the nucleus.
- ☐ b) neutrons in the nucleus.
- ☐ c) electrons in the outer shells.
- ☐ d) a, b, and c are all correct.

9 The number and arrangement of electrons in an atom's outer energy level determine the atom's
- ☐ a) atomic weight.
- ☐ b) atomic number.
- ☐ c) molecular weight.
- ☐ d) chemical properties.

10 A _____ is a quantity with a weight in grams equal to an element's atomic weight.
- ☐ a) mole
- ☐ b) molecule
- ☐ c) compound
- ☐ d) synthesis

11 Energy in motion is called
- ☐ a) end product.
- ☐ b) kinetic.
- ☐ c) transfer work.
- ☐ d) potential.

12 All organic compounds in the human body contain all of the following elements except
- ☐ a) hydrogen.
- ☐ b) oxygen.
- ☐ c) carbon.
- ☐ d) calcium.

13 All the chemical reactions that occur in the human body are collectively referred to as

- ☐ a) anabolism.
- ☐ b) catabolism.
- ☐ c) metabolism.
- ☐ d) homeostasis.

14 A pH of 7.8 in the human body typifies a condition referred to as

- ☐ a) acidosis.
- ☐ b) alkalosis.
- ☐ c) dehydration.
- ☐ d) homeostasis.

15 A(n) _____ is a solute that dissociates to release hydrogen ions, and a(n) _____ is a solute that removes hydrogen ions from solution.

- ☐ a) base, acid
- ☐ b) salt, base
- ☐ c) acid, salt
- ☐ d) acid, base

16 Special organic catalysts that control chemical reactions in the human body are called

- ☐ a) enzymes.
- ☐ b) cytozymes.
- ☐ c) cofactors.
- ☐ d) activators.
- ☐ e) cytochromes.

17 Complementary base pairing in DNA includes the pairs

- ☐ a) adenine–uracil and cytosine–guanine.
- ☐ b) adenine–thymine and cytosine–guanine.
- ☐ c) adenine–guanine and cytosine–thymine.
- ☐ d) guanine–uracil and cytosine–thymine.

18 When the energy stored in ATP is released, it is broken down into

- ☐ a) adenosine + energy.
- ☐ b) AMP + P + energy.
- ☐ c) P + P + P + energy.
- ☐ d) ADP + P + energy.

Short answer

19 What are the three stable subatomic particles in atoms?

_____

_____

_____

20 What four major classes of organic compounds are found in the body?

_____

_____

_____

21 List three functions performed by lipids in the body.

_____

_____

_____

22 Identify the structural characteristics of a protein.

_____

_____

_____

23 a) What three components make up a nucleotide of DNA?
b) What three components make up a nucleotide of RNA?

_____

_____

_____

24 Explain how enzymes function in chemical reactions.

_____

_____

_____

25 What is a salt? How does a salt differ from an acid or a base?

_____

_____

_____

26 Explain the differences among nonpolar covalent bonds, polar covalent bonds, and ionic bonds.

_____

_____

_____

27 An organic molecule has the following constituents: carbon, hydrogen, oxygen, nitrogen, and phosphorus. Is the molecule more likely to be a carbohydrate, a lipid, a protein, or a nucleic acid?

_____

_____

_____

28 Explain how an insect can walk across the top of a pond without falling through the surface.

_____

_____

_____

29 A student eats a dinner of tomato salad with vinegar dressing and a glass of wine. Shortly thereafter he complains of an upset stomach. Considering what you know about pH and foods, can you predict why his stomach is upset? Could you give any suggestions as to the kinds of foods he could eat to alleviate his symptoms?

_____

_____

_____

Sketching exercise

30 An oxygen atom has eight protons. a) Sketch in the arrangement of electrons around the nucleus of the oxygen atom. b) How many more electrons will it take to fill the outermost energy level?

Oxygen atom

Vocabulary

In the space provided, write the boldfaced terms introduced in this section that contain the indicated word part.

1 glycos- *(sugar)*

2 aero- *(air)*

3 micro- *(small)*

4 lyso- *(a loosening)*

1 _____

2 _____

3 _____

4 _____

Short answer

Correctly label the indicated structures on the cell diagram below, and describe the functions of each.

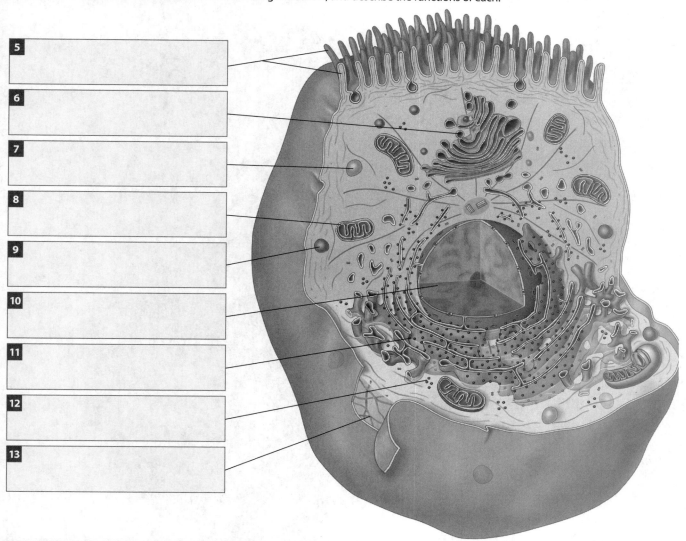

5

6

7

8

9

10

11

12

13

Section integration

What is the advantage of having some of the cellular organelles enclosed by a membrane similar to the plasma membrane?

14 _____

Vocabulary

In the space provided, write the boldfaced terms introduced in this section that contain the indicated word part.

1 glycos- *(sugar)*

2 aero- *(air)*

3 micro- *(small)*

4 lyso- *(a loosening)*

1 _____

2 _____

3 _____

4 _____

Short answer

Correctly label the indicated structures on the cell diagram below, and describe the functions of each.

5

6

7

8

9

10

11

12

13

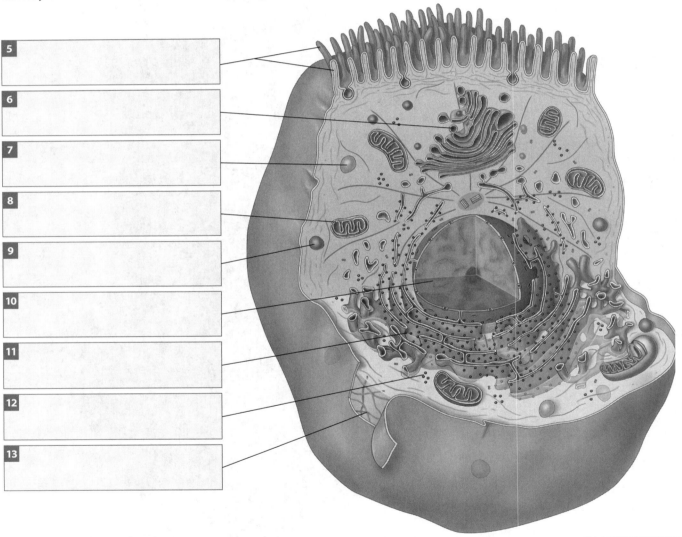

Section integration

What is the advantage of having some of the cellular organelles enclosed by a membrane similar to the plasma membrane?

14 _____

Matching

Match each lettered term with the most closely related description.

a. introns
b. transcription
c. tRNA
d. chromosomes
e. exons
f. genetic information
g. nucleus
h. thymine
i. mRNA
j. gene
k. uracil
l. nuclear envelope
m. nuclear pore
n. nucleoli

1	DNA strands and histones	1
2	DNA nitrogenous base	2
3	Double membrane	3
4	mRNA noncoding regions	4
5	RNA nitrogenous base	5
6	Assemble ribosomal subunits	6
7	Passageway for functional mRNA	7
8	mRNA formation	8
9	Functional unit of heredity	9
10	mRNA coding regions	10
11	Codon	11
12	Anticodon	12
13	Cell control center	13
14	DNA nucleotide sequence	14

Short answer

The sequence of DNA bases at right are from a protein-coding gene. Use the sequence as the basis for answering the following questions.

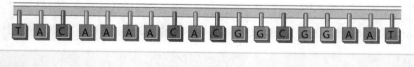

T A C A A A A C A C G G C G G A A T

15 Provide the corresponding mRNA base sequence, and insert a slash mark (/) between the codons.

16 Convert the mRNA codons you decoded above into tRNA anticodons.

15 _____

16 _____

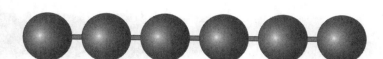

17 Using the genetic code table in Module 3.10, translate the anticodon sequence into the amino acid sequence of this polypeptide.

17 _____

Section integration

The nucleus is often described as the control center of the cell. Explain the role of the nucleus in maintaining homeostasis.

18 _____

Matching

Match each lettered term with the most closely related description.

a. introns
b. transcription
c. tRNA
d. chromosomes
e. exons
f. genetic information
g. nucleus
h. thymine
i. mRNA
j. gene
k. uracil
l. nuclear envelope
m. nuclear pore
n. nucleoli

1	DNA strands and histones
2	DNA nitrogenous base
3	Double membrane
4	mRNA noncoding regions
5	RNA nitrogenous base
6	Assemble ribosomal subunits
7	Passageway for functional mRNA
8	mRNA formation
9	Functional unit of heredity
10	mRNA coding regions
11	Codon
12	Anticodon
13	Cell control center
14	DNA nucleotide sequence

1 _____
2 _____
3 _____
4 _____
5 _____
6 _____
7 _____
8 _____
9 _____
10 _____
11 _____
12 _____
13 _____
14 _____

Short answer

The sequence of DNA bases at right are from a protein-coding gene. Use the sequence as the basis for answering the following questions.

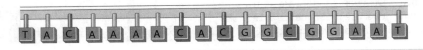

T A C A A A A C A C G G C G G A A T

15 Provide the corresponding mRNA base sequence, and insert a slash mark (/) between the codons.

15 _____

16 Convert the mRNA codons you decoded above into tRNA anticodons.

16 _____

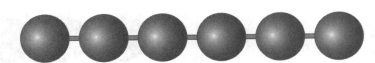

17 Using the genetic code table in Module 3.10, translate the anticodon sequence into the amino acid sequence of this polypeptide.

17 _____

Section integration

The nucleus is often described as the control center of the cell. Explain the role of the nucleus in maintaining homeostasis.

18 _____
_____

Concept map

Use each of the following terms once to fill in the blank boxes to correctly complete the map.

- exocytosis
- diffusion
- "cell eating"
- molecular size
- pinocytosis
- facilitated diffusion
- vesicular transport
- net diffusion of water
- active transport
- specificity

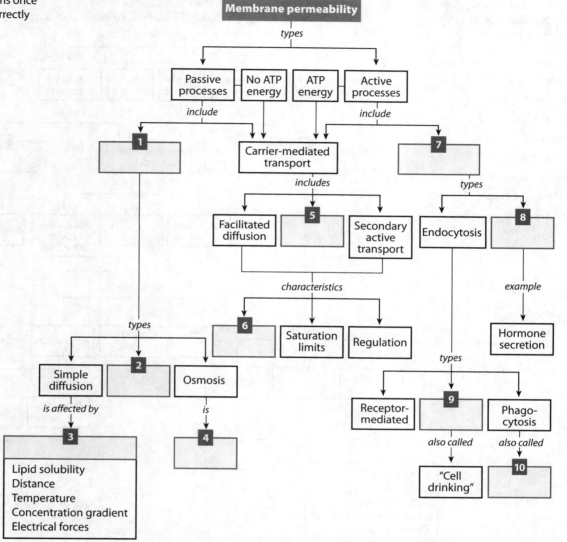

Short answer

Classify each of the following situations as an example of diffusion, osmosis, or neither.

11 You walk into a room and smell a balsam-scented candle.

12 Water flows through a garden hose.

13 Grass in the yard wilts after being exposed to excess chemical fertilizer.

14 A sugar cube placed in a cup of hot tea dissolves.

15 After soaking several hours in water containing sodium chloride, a stalk of celery weighs less than before it was placed in the salty water.

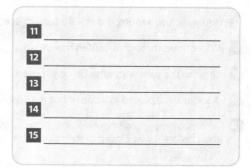

Concept map

Use each of the following terms once to fill in the blank boxes to correctly complete the map.

- exocytosis
- diffusion
- "cell eating"
- molecular size
- pinocytosis
- facilitated diffusion
- vesicular transport
- net diffusion of water
- active transport
- specificity

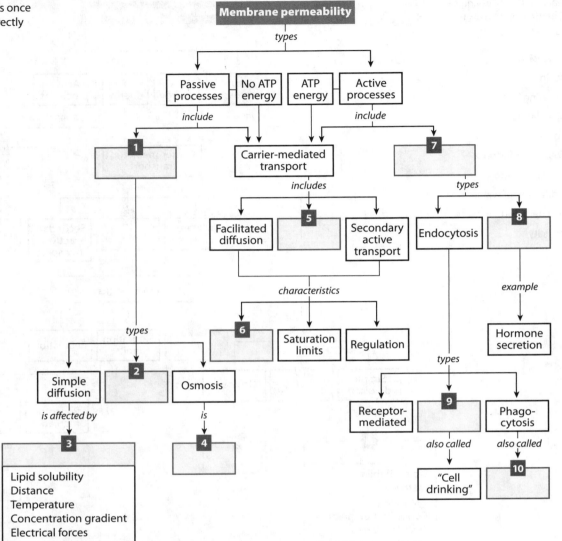

Short answer

Classify each of the following situations as an example of diffusion, osmosis, or neither.

11 You walk into a room and smell a balsam-scented candle.

12 Water flows through a garden hose.

13 Grass in the yard wilts after being exposed to excess chemical fertilizer.

14 A sugar cube placed in a cup of hot tea dissolves.

15 After soaking several hours in water containing sodium chloride, a stalk of celery weighs less than before it was placed in the salty water.

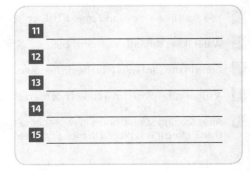

Concept map

Use each of the following terms once to fill in the blank boxes to correctly complete the map.

- metaphase
- DNA replication
- somatic cells
- G$_2$ phase
- telophase
- mitosis
- cytokinesis
- G$_1$ phase

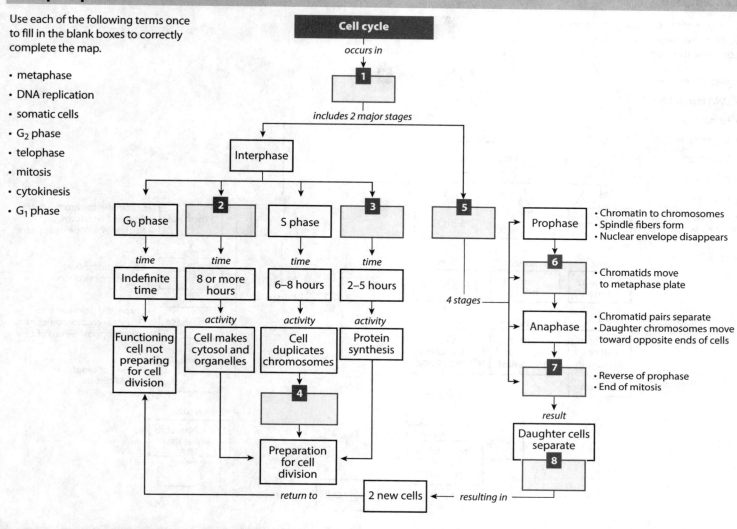

Cell cycle

occurs in

1

includes 2 major stages

Interphase

2 | S phase | **3** | **5** | Prophase
- Chromatin to chromosomes
- Spindle fibers form
- Nuclear envelope disappears

G$_0$ phase

time

Indefinite time | 8 or more hours | 6–8 hours | 2–5 hours

4 stages

6
- Chromatids move to metaphase plate

activity

Functioning cell not preparing for cell division | Cell makes cytosol and organelles | Cell duplicates chromosomes | Protein synthesis

Anaphase
- Chromatid pairs separate
- Daughter chromosomes move toward opposite ends of cells

4

7
- Reverse of prophase
- End of mitosis

Preparation for cell division

result

Daughter cells separate

8

return to — 2 new cells ← *resulting in*

Vocabulary

In the space provided, write the boldfaced terms introduced in this section that contain the indicated word part.

9 telo- *(end)*   **9** _____

10 pro- *(before)*   **10** _____

11 centro- *(in the middle)*   **11** _____

Section integration

The muscle cells that that make up skeletal muscle tissue are large and multinucleated. They form early in development as groups of embryonic cells fuse together, contributing their nuclei and losing their individual plasma membranes. Describe an alternate mechanism that would also result in a large, multinucleated cell.

12 _____

_____

Concept map

Use each of the following terms once to fill in the blank boxes to correctly complete the map.

- metaphase
- DNA replication
- somatic cells
- G_2 phase
- telophase
- mitosis
- cytokinesis
- G_1 phase

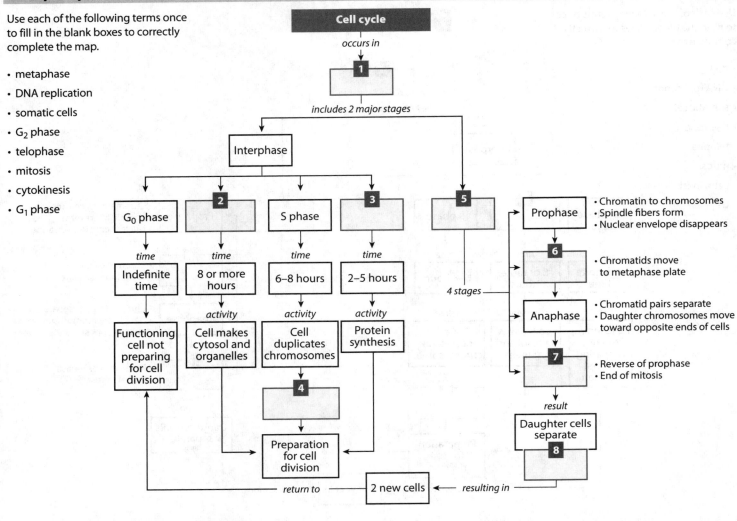

Cell cycle

occurs in

1

includes 2 major stages

Interphase

2 | **3** | **5**

G_0 phase | S phase

time
Indefinite time | 8 or more hours | 6–8 hours | 2–5 hours

activity
Functioning cell not preparing for cell division | Cell makes cytosol and organelles | Cell duplicates chromosomes | Protein synthesis

4

Preparation for cell division

return to — **2 new cells** ← *resulting in*

4 stages

Prophase
- Chromatin to chromosomes
- Spindle fibers form
- Nuclear envelope disappears

6
- Chromatids move to metaphase plate

Anaphase
- Chromatid pairs separate
- Daughter chromosomes move toward opposite ends of cells

7
- Reverse of prophase
- End of mitosis

result
Daughter cells separate

8

Vocabulary

In the space provided, write the boldfaced terms introduced in this section that contain the indicated word part.

9 telo- *(end)*

10 pro- *(before)*

11 centro- *(in the middle)*

9 _____

10 _____

11 _____

Section integration

The muscle cells that that make up skeletal muscle tissue are large and multinucleated. They form early in development as groups of embryonic cells fuse together, contributing their nuclei and losing their individual plasma membranes. Describe an alternate mechanism that would also result in a large, multinucleated cell.

12 _____

_____

Chapter Review Questions

Multiple choice

Select the correct answer from the list provided.

1 Which of the following is *not* a characteristic of the cell theory?
- a) Cells are the building blocks of life.
- b) Cells combine to form tissues.
- c) All new cells come from the division of pre-existing cells.
- d) Cells are the smallest units that perform all vital physiological functions.

2 The process of gradual cell specialization is called
- a) fertilization.
- b) meiosis.
- c) differentiation.
- d) metastasis.

3 The _____ is/are responsible for producing 95 percent of the ATP required by the cell.
- a) Golgi apparatus
- b) mitochondria
- c) rough endoplasmic reticulum
- d) smooth endoplasmic reticulum

4 Somatic cell nuclei contain _____ pairs of chromosomes.
- a) 8
- b) 23
- c) 46
- d) 92

5 The construction of a functional polypeptide by using the information in an mRNA strand is called
- a) translation.
- b) transcription.
- c) replication.
- d) differentiation.

6 Genetically controlled cell death is called
- a) mitosis.
- b) apoptosis.
- c) metastasis.
- d) mutation.

7 The _____ phase of protein synthesis encodes genetic instructions on a strand of mRNA.
- a) transcription
- b) translation
- c) transmigration
- d) transference

8 When substances pass through the plasma membrane by active processes, which molecule is required?
- a) RNA polymerase
- b) ATP
- c) DNA
- d) tRNA

9 The sodium–potassium exchange pump
- a) is an example of facilitated diffusion.
- b) does not require the input of cellular energy in the form of ATP.
- c) moves the sodium and potassium ions along their concentration gradients.
- d) is composed of a carrier protein located in the plasma membrane.

10 If a cell lacked ribosomes it would not be able to
- a) produce complex carbohydrates.
- b) synthesize proteins.
- c) divide.
- d) produce ATP.

11 Suppose a DNA segment has the following nucleotide sequence: CTC/ATA/CGA/TTC/AAG/TTA. Which nucleotide sequence would a complementary mRNA strand have?
- a) GAG/UAU/GAU/AAC/UUG/AAU
- b) GAG/TAT/GCT/AAG/TTC/AAT
- c) GAG/UAU/GCU/AAG/UUC/AAU
- d) GUG/UAU/GGA/UUG/AAG/GGU

12 How many amino acids are coded in the DNA segment in the previous question?
- a) 18
- b) 9
- c) 6
- d) 3

13 Identify the five functional classes of membrane proteins.

_____

_____

_____

14 Distinguish between mitosis and cytokinesis.

_____

_____

_____

15 Differentiate between diffusion and osmosis.

_____

_____

_____

16 Which organelle contains its own DNA, and what does it code for?

_____

_____

_____

17 List the nonmembranous organelles and then list the membranous organelles.

_____

_____

_____

18 List the stages of mitosis, and for each stage briefly describe the events that occur.

_____

_____

_____

19 If a cell had microvilli on its plasma membrane, in which activity is it likely to be actively engaged?

_____

_____

_____

20 If a red blood cell were immersed in a hypotonic solution, in which direction would water flow, and what effect would it have on the cell?

_____

_____

_____

21 Order the following steps of protein synthesis into the proper sequence:

a) mRNA exits nucleus through nuclear pore;

b) introns are snipped from mRNA;

c) amino acids form peptide bonds;

d) ribosomal subunits detach from mRNA;

e) transcription of DNA forms mRNA;

f) tRNA anticodons bind to mRNA codons;

g) ribosomal subunits bind to mRNA

_____

22 Describe the steps involved in phagocytosis.

_____

_____

_____

23 Why does mitosis produce cells containing 46 chromosomes, whereas meiosis produces cells containing only 23 chromosomes?

_____

_____

_____

24 Steroid hormones such as estrogen and testosterone are lipid molecules. Explain how these molecules cross the plasma membrane and enter the cell.

_____

_____

_____

25 Describe the process used by malignant tumors to accelerate their growth.

_____

_____

_____

Labeling

Label the types of epithelial tissues shown in the drawing to the right.

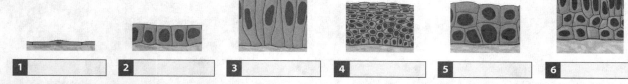

| 1 | | 2 | | 3 | | 4 | | 5 | | 6 | |

Concept map

Use the following terms once to fill in the blank boxes to correctly complete the map.

- endocrine glands
- ducts
- mucous cells
- apocrine secretion
- interstitial fluid
- mucus
- merocrine secretion
- epithelial surfaces
- mucin
- exocrine glands
- holocrine secretion

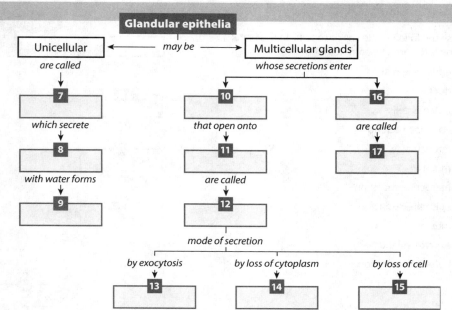

Vocabulary

Write the term for each of the following descriptions in the space provided.

18 A term meaning no blood vessels

19 A gland whose glandular cells form sac-like pockets

20 A type of epithelium that withstands stretching and that changes in appearance as stretching occurs

21 The cell junction formed by the partial fusion of the lipid portions of two plasma membranes

22 The complex structure attached to the basal surface of an epithelium

23 A gland that has a single duct

24 The type of epithelium lining the pericardial, pleural, and peritoneal body cavities

18 _____
19 _____
20 _____
21 _____
22 _____
23 _____
24 _____

Short answer

Fill in the missing epithelium type or structure.

Type of Epithelium	Structure (or Organ)
25	Lining of the trachea
Transitional epithelium	26
27	Surface of the skin
28	Lining of the small intestine

Type of Epithelium	Structure (or Organ)
Simple squamous epithelium	29
Cuboidal epithelium	30
31	Ducts of sweat glands

Labeling

Label the types of epithelial tissues shown in the drawing to the right.

 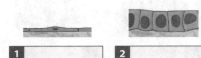 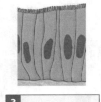   

| 1 | 2 | 3 | 4 | 5 | 6 |

Concept map

Use the following terms once to fill in the blank boxes to correctly complete the map.

- endocrine glands
- ducts
- mucous cells
- apocrine secretion
- interstitial fluid
- mucus
- merocrine secretion
- epithelial surfaces
- mucin
- exocrine glands
- holocrine secretion

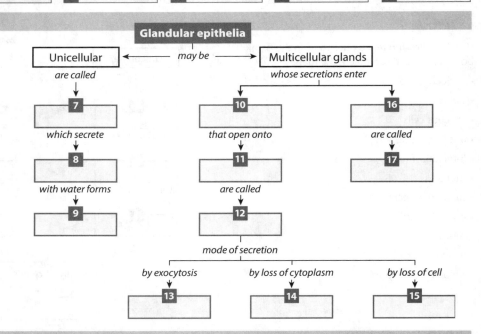

Vocabulary

Write the term for each of the following descriptions in the space provided.

18 A term meaning no blood vessels

19 A gland whose glandular cells form sac-like pockets

20 A type of epithelium that withstands stretching and that changes in appearance as stretching occurs

21 The cell junction formed by the partial fusion of the lipid portions of two plasma membranes

22 The complex structure attached to the basal surface of an epithelium

23 A gland that has a single duct

24 The type of epithelium lining the pericardial, pleural, and peritoneal body cavities

18 _____
19 _____
20 _____
21 _____
22 _____
23 _____
24 _____

Short answer

Fill in the missing epithelium type or structure.

Type of Epithelium	Structure (or Organ)
25	Lining of the trachea
Transitional epithelium	26
27	Surface of the skin
28	Lining of the small intestine

Type of Epithelium	Structure (or Organ)
Simple squamous epithelium	29
Cuboidal epithelium	30
31	Ducts of sweat glands

Concept map

Use the following terms once to fill in the blank boxes to correctly complete the map.

- loose connective tissue
- chondrocytes in lacunae
- fluid connective tissue
- tendons
- ligaments
- regular
- hyaline
- blood
- adipose
- bone

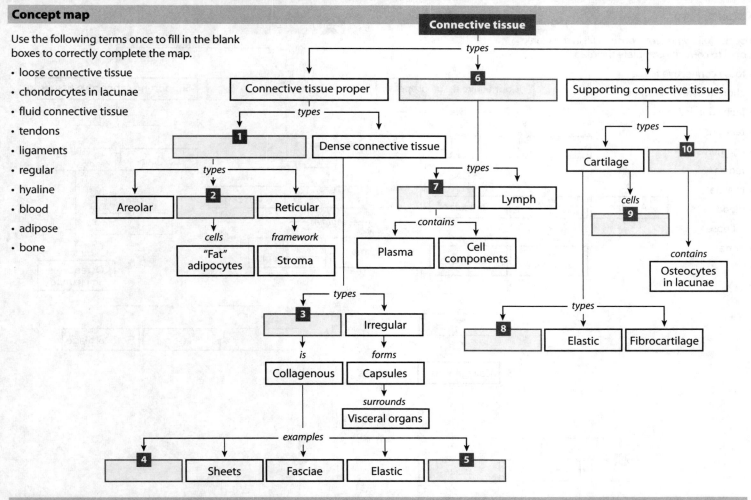

Vocabulary

In the space provided, write the boldfaced terms introduced in this section that contain the indicated word part.

11 peri- *(around)*

12 os- *(bone)*

13 chondro- *(cartilage)*

14 inter- *(between)*

15 lacus- *(lake)*

11 _____

12 _____

13 _____

14 _____

15 _____

Enter the appropriate term for each description below.

16 A cartilage cell

17 Bone tissue

18 A type of cartilage that has a matrix with little ground substance and large amounts of collagen fibers

19 Cells that store lipid reserves

20 The membrane that lines freely movable joint cavities

21 The membrane that covers the surface of the body

22 Separates cartilage from surrounding tissues

16 _____

17 _____

18 _____

19 _____

20 _____

21 _____

22 _____

Concept map

Use the following terms once to fill in the blank boxes to correctly complete the map.

- loose connective tissue
- chondrocytes in lacunae
- fluid connective tissue
- tendons
- ligaments
- regular
- hyaline
- blood
- adipose
- bone

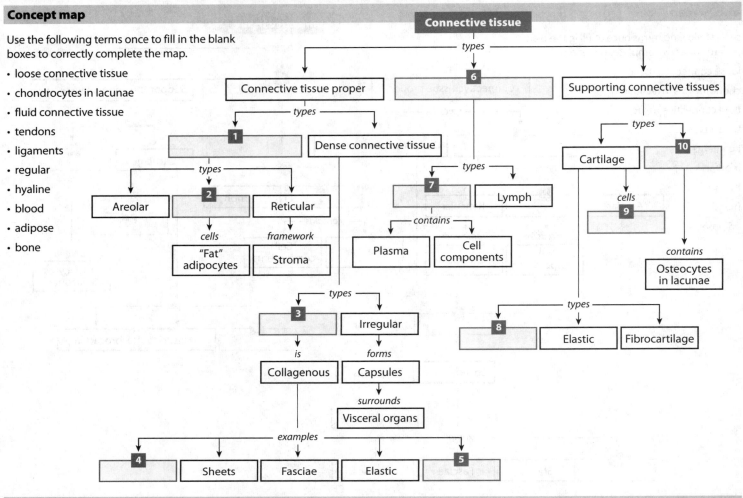

Vocabulary

In the space provided, write the boldfaced terms introduced in this section that contain the indicated word part.

11 peri- *(around)*   **11** _____

12 os- *(bone)*   **12** _____

13 chondro- *(cartilage)* **13** _____

14 inter- *(between)*   **14** _____

15 lacus- *(lake)*   **15** _____

Enter the appropriate term for each description below.

16 A cartilage cell

17 Bone tissue

18 A type of cartilage that has a matrix with little ground substance and large amounts of collagen fibers

19 Cells that store lipid reserves

20 The membrane that lines freely movable joint cavities

21 The membrane that covers the surface of the body

22 Separates cartilage from surrounding tissues

16 _____

17 _____

18 _____

19 _____

20 _____

21 _____

22 _____

Concept map

Complete the concept maps using key terms and concepts covered in this section.

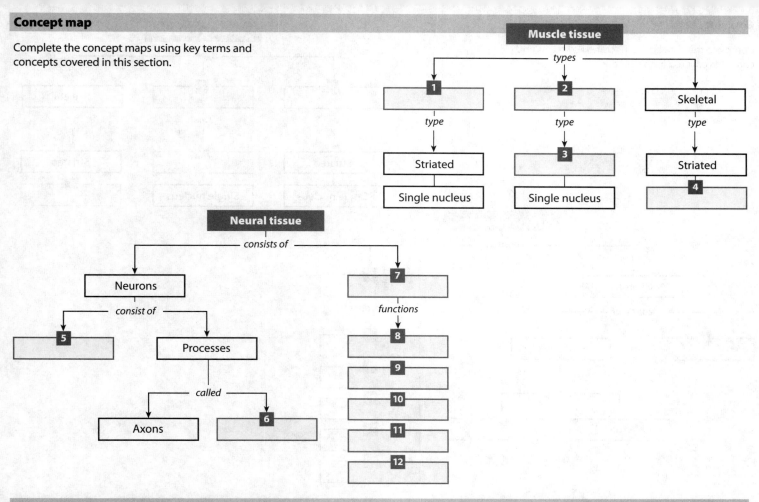

Vocabulary

Write the term for each of the following descriptions in the space provided.

13 A single structure that extends from the cell body of a neuron and carries information to other cells

14 A specialized intercellular junction between cardiac muscle cells

15 The supporting cells found in neural tissue

16 Muscle tissue that contains large, multinucleate, striated cells

17 Muscle tissue that regulates the diameter of blood vessels and respiratory passageways

18 The repair process that occurs after inflammation has subsided

19 The first process in a tissue's response to injury

13 _____

14 _____

15 _____

16 _____

17 _____

18 _____

19 _____

Section integration

During inflammation, both blood flow and blood vessel permeability increase in the injured area.
Describe how these responses aid the cleanup process and eliminate the inflammatory stimuli in the injured area.

20 _____

_____

Concept map

Complete the concept maps using key terms and concepts covered in this section.

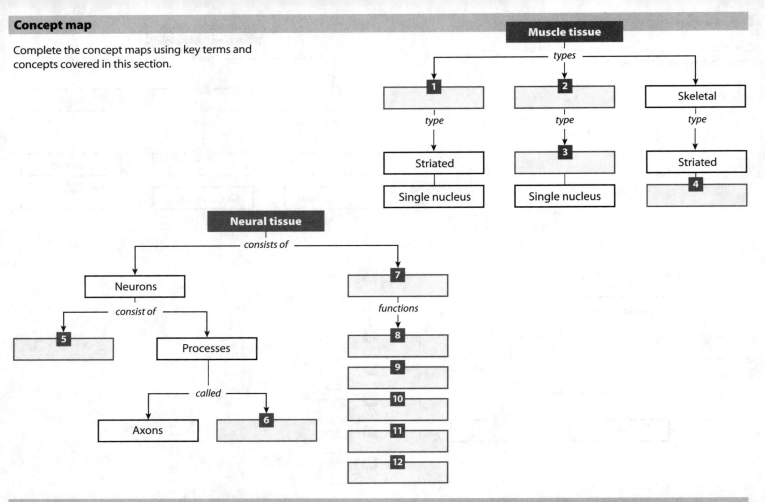

Muscle tissue

types

1 → type → Striated → Single nucleus

2 → type → 3 → Single nucleus

Skeletal → type → Striated → 4

Neural tissue

consists of

Neurons → consist of → 5 , Processes → called → Axons , 6

7 → functions → 8 , 9 , 10 , 11 , 12

Vocabulary

Write the term for each of the following descriptions in the space provided.

13 A single structure that extends from the cell body of a neuron and carries information to other cells

13 _____

14 A specialized intercellular junction between cardiac muscle cells

14 _____

15 The supporting cells found in neural tissue

15 _____

16 Muscle tissue that contains large, multinucleate, striated cells

16 _____

17 Muscle tissue that regulates the diameter of blood vessels and respiratory passageways

17 _____

18 The repair process that occurs after inflammation has subsided

18 _____

19 The first process in a tissue's response to injury

19 _____

Section integration

During inflammation, both blood flow and blood vessel permeability increase in the injured area.
Describe how these responses aid the cleanup process and eliminate the inflammatory stimuli in the injured area.

20 _____

_____

Chapter Review Questions

Labeling

Identify the three categories of cartilage shown below.

1	2	3

Identify the three categories of muscle shown below.

4	5	6

Identify the six connective tissue types shown below.

7	8	9	10	11	12

Multiple choice

Select the correct answer from the list provided.

13 Tissue that is specialized for contraction is
- [ ] a) epithelial tissue.
- [ ] b) connective tissue.
- [ ] c) muscle tissue.
- [ ] d) neural tissue.

14 The specialized intercellular junctions found in cardiac muscle are
- [ ] a) hemidesmosomes.
- [ ] b) intercalated discs.
- [ ] c) desmosomes.
- [ ] d) microvilli.

15 Collections of specialized cells and cell products that perform a limited number of functions are called
- [ ] a) cellular aggregates.
- [ ] b) organs.
- [ ] c) tissues.
- [ ] d) organ systems.

16 Axons, dendrites, and a cell body are characteristic of cells located in
- [ ] a) neural tissue.
- [ ] b) connective tissue.
- [ ] c) muscle tissue.
- [ ] d) epithelial tissue.

17 Specialized cells, extracellular protein fibers, and ground substance are characteristic of which type of tissue?
- [ ] a) muscle tissue
- [ ] b) epithelial tissue
- [ ] c) neural tissue
- [ ] d) connective tissue

18 Which of the following epithelia most easily permits diffusion?
- [ ] a) stratified squamous epithelium
- [ ] b) simple squamous epithelium
- [ ] c) transitional epithelium
- [ ] d) simple columnar epithelium

19 The tissue lining the peritoneal cavity is an example of a
- [ ] a) mucous membrane.
- [ ] b) serous membrane.
- [ ] c) cutaneous membrane.
- [ ] d) synovial membrane.

20 The addition of new layers of cartilage to the outer surface is which of the following types of growth?
- [ ] a) appositional
- [ ] b) interstitial

21 Which of the following is the most common form of connective tissue proper?
- [ ] a) reticular tissue
- [ ] b) areolar tissue
- [ ] c) adipose tissue
- [ ] d) elastic tissue

22 Which of the following membranes line movable joints?
- [ ] a) mucous membranes
- [ ] b) serous membranes
- [ ] c) cutaneous membranes
- [ ] d) synovial membranes

Short answer

23 Why is stratified squamous epithelium well suited to form the surface of the skin and the lining of the mouth and throat?

_____
_____
_____

24 Differentiate between endocrine glands and exocrine glands.

_____
_____
_____

25 Which two cell populations make up neural tissue? What is the function of each?

_____
_____
_____

26 Why are infections always a serious threat after a severe skin burn or abrasion?

_____
_____
_____

27 Describe the unique characteristics you would expect to see when examining cardiac muscle tissue under a light microscope.

_____
_____
_____

28 During a lab practical, Jason examines a tissue that is composed of densely packed protein fibers that are running parallel. There are no striations, but small nuclei are visible. Jason identifies the tissue as skeletal muscle. Why is Jason's choice wrong, and which tissue is he probably observing?

_____
_____
_____

29 While jogging through campus, Emily trips off a curb and falls onto the street. Her hands and exposed knees slide across the rough asphalt, resulting in deep abrasions. Outline the tissue injury response Emily's body will undergo.

_____
_____
_____

Concept map

Use each of the following terms once to fill in the blank boxes to correctly complete the map.

- accessory structures
- collagen
- connective
- epidermis
- fat
- granulosum
- hypodermis
- nerves
- papillary layer
- reticular layer

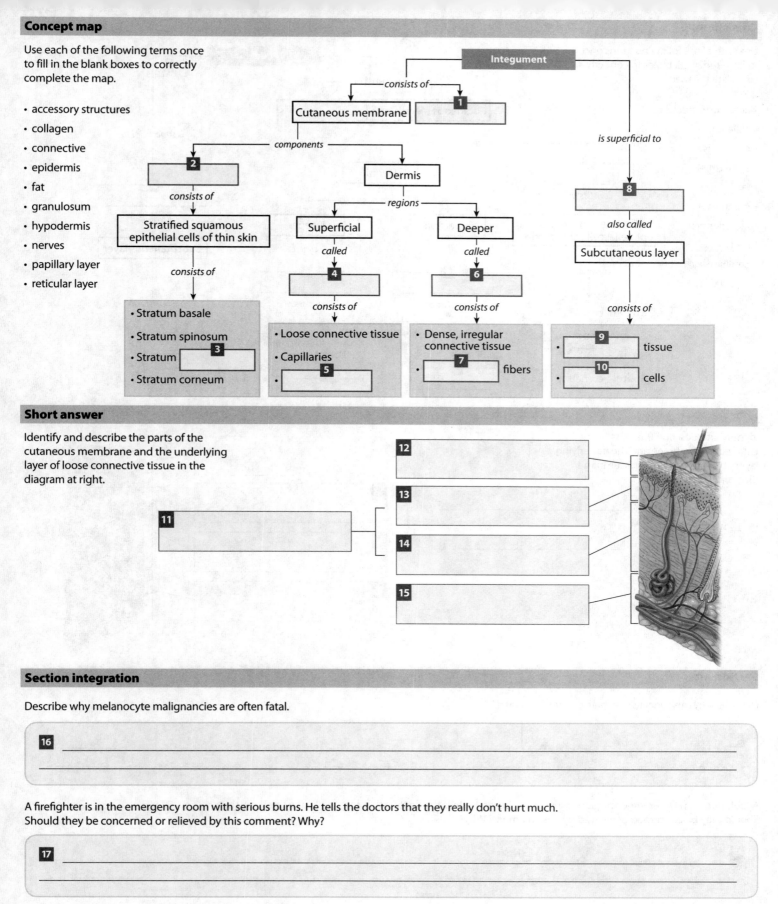

Integument

consists of

Cutaneous membrane | **1**

components

2

consists of

Stratified squamous epithelial cells of thin skin

consists of

- Stratum basale
- Stratum spinosum
- Stratum **3**
- Stratum corneum

Dermis

regions

Superficial | Deeper

called | *called*

4 | **6**

consists of | *consists of*

- Loose connective tissue
- Capillaries
- **5**

- Dense, irregular connective tissue
- **7** fibers

is superficial to

8

also called

Subcutaneous layer

consists of

- **9** tissue
- **10** cells

Short answer

Identify and describe the parts of the cutaneous membrane and the underlying layer of loose connective tissue in the diagram at right.

11

12

13

14

15

Section integration

Describe why melanocyte malignancies are often fatal.

16 _____

_____

A firefighter is in the emergency room with serious burns. He tells the doctors that they really don't hurt much. Should they be concerned or relieved by this comment? Why?

17 _____

_____

Concept map

Use each of the following terms once to fill in the blank boxes to correctly complete the map.

- accessory structures
- collagen
- connective
- epidermis
- fat
- granulosum
- hypodermis
- nerves
- papillary layer
- reticular layer

Integument

consists of

Cutaneous membrane | **1**

components

2

Dermis

is superficial to

8

consists of

Stratified squamous epithelial cells of thin skin

regions

Superficial

Deeper

also called

Subcutaneous layer

called

4

called

6

consists of

- Stratum basale
- Stratum spinosum
- Stratum **3**
- Stratum corneum

consists of

- Loose connective tissue
- Capillaries
- **5**

consists of

- Dense, irregular connective tissue
- **7** fibers

consists of

- **9** tissue
- **10** cells

Short answer

Identify and describe the parts of the cutaneous membrane and the underlying layer of loose connective tissue in the diagram at right.

11

12

13

14

15

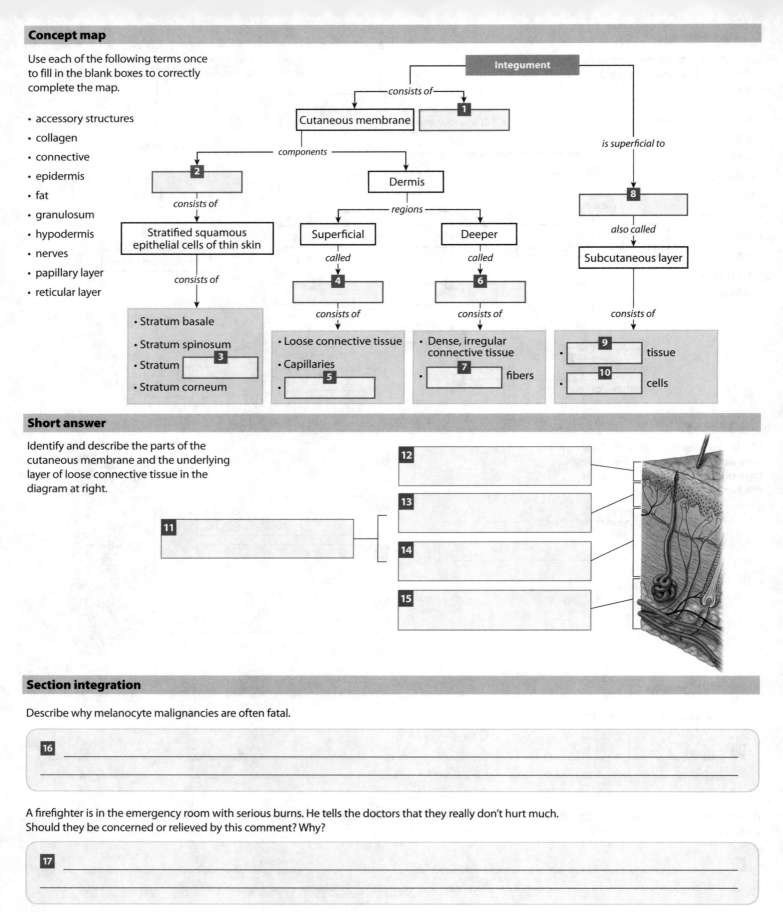

Section integration

Describe why melanocyte malignancies are often fatal.

16

A firefighter is in the emergency room with serious burns. He tells the doctors that they really don't hurt much. Should they be concerned or relieved by this comment? Why?

17

Labeling

Label the structures of a typical nail in the accompanying figures.

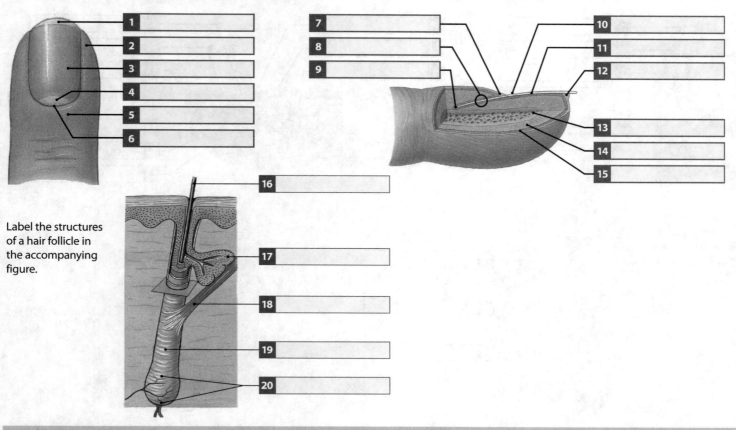

1	
2	
3	
4	
5	
6	

7	
8	
9	

10	
11	
12	
13	
14	
15	

| 16 | |

Label the structures of a hair follicle in the accompanying figure.

17	
18	
19	
20	

Matching

Match each lettered term with the most closely related description.

a. malignant melanoma

b. keloid

c. nail root

d. sebum

e. apocrine sweat glands

f. eponychium

g. EGF

h. vitamin D_3

i. reticular layer of dermis

j. merocrine sweat glands

21	Produced by epidermal cells stimulated by UV radiation	21	_____
22	Epithelial fold not visible from the surface	22	_____
23	Found in the armpit	23	_____
24	Peptide produced by salivary glands	24	_____
25	Site of hair production	25	_____
26	Excessive scar tissue	26	_____
27	Oily lipid secretion	27	_____
28	Melanocytes metastasize through the lymphatic system	28	_____
29	Abundant in the palms and soles	29	_____
30	Cuticle	30	_____

Section integration

Many people change the natural appearance of their hair, either by coloring it or by altering the degree of curl in it. Which layers of the hair do you suppose are affected by the chemicals added during these procedures? Why are the effects of the procedures not permanent?

| 31 | _____ |

Labeling

Label the structures of a typical nail in the accompanying figures.

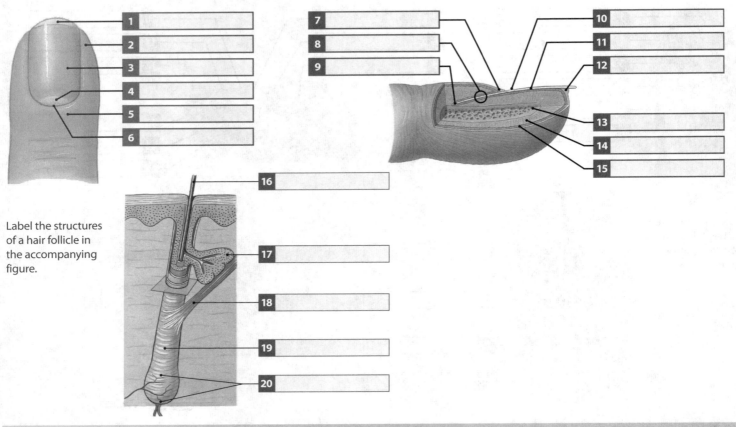

1	
2	
3	
4	
5	
6	

7	
8	
9	

10	
11	
12	
13	
14	
15	

Label the structures of a hair follicle in the accompanying figure.

16	
17	
18	
19	
20	

Matching

Match each lettered term with the most closely related description.

a. malignant melanoma

b. keloid

c. nail root

d. sebum

e. apocrine sweat glands

f. eponychium

g. EGF

h. vitamin D₃

i. reticular layer of dermis

j. merocrine sweat glands

21	Produced by epidermal cells stimulated by UV radiation
22	Epithelial fold not visible from the surface
23	Found in the armpit
24	Peptide produced by salivary glands
25	Site of hair production
26	Excessive scar tissue
27	Oily lipid secretion
28	Melanocytes metastasize through the lymphatic system
29	Abundant in the palms and soles
30	Cuticle

21	_____
22	_____
23	_____
24	_____
25	_____
26	_____
27	_____
28	_____
29	_____
30	_____

Section integration

Many people change the natural appearance of their hair, either by coloring it or by altering the degree of curl in it. Which layers of the hair do you suppose are affected by the chemicals added during these procedures? Why are the effects of the procedures not permanent?

31 _____

Chapter Review Questions

Labeling

Identify the layers of the epidermis in this image.

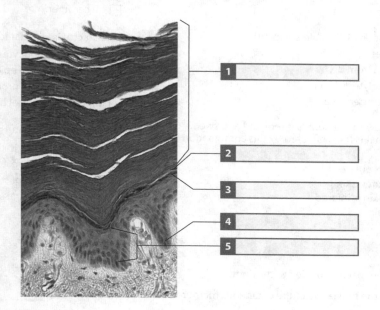

1 _____
2 _____
3 _____
4 _____
5 _____

True/False

Indicate whether each statement is true or false.

6 Wrinkles and sagging skin are caused by damage to collagen fibers due to aging and exposure to ultraviolet radiation.

7 Another name for the hypodermis is the subcutaneous layer.

8 The perspiration you experience during intense exercise is called insensible perspiration.

9 The dermis is dominated by adipose tissue and therefore is an important site for energy storage.

10 Lamellated (pacinian) corpuscles are sensitive to deep pressure.

11 Bluish skin as a result of decreased oxygen in blood is called cyanosis.

12 The root hair plexus is a smooth muscle whose contraction pulls on the follicle, forcing the hair to stand erect.

13 The primary pigments involved in skin coloration are carotene and melanin.

6 _____
7 _____
8 _____
9 _____
10 _____
11 _____
12 _____
13 _____

Multiple choice

Select the correct answer from the list provided.

14 Which portion of the hair follicle produces the hair?
- ☐ a) hair shaft
- ☐ b) hair matrix
- ☐ c) hair root plexus
- ☐ d) arrector pili

15 Which of the following glands discharges an oily secretion that coats the hair and the adjacent surface of the skin?
- ☐ a) apocrine gland
- ☐ b) sebaceous gland
- ☐ c) merocrine gland
- ☐ d) sweat gland

16 Fine touch, pressure, and vibrations are perceived by which nerve endings?

- ☐ a) free nerve endings
- ☐ b) Meissner's corpuscles
- ☐ c) tactile discs
- ☐ d) Ruffini corpuscles

17 What is the primary function of sensible perspiration?

- ☐ a) to get rid of wastes
- ☐ b) to protect the skin from dryness
- ☐ c) to maintain electrolyte balance
- ☐ d) to reduce body temperature

18 In the elderly, blood supply to the dermis is reduced and sweat glands are less active. What is most affected by this combination of factors?

- ☐ a) ability to thermoregulate
- ☐ b) ability to heal injured skin
- ☐ c) ease with which skin is injured
- ☐ d) ability to grow hair

19 Which term is applied to the stratum corneum of the nail root that extends over the exposed nail?

- ☐ a) hyponychium
- ☐ b) eponychium
- ☐ c) lunula
- ☐ d) cerumen

20 Which factor is associated with darker skin color?

- ☐ a) more melanocytes present in skin
- ☐ b) more layers of epidermis
- ☐ c) more melanin produced by melanocytes
- ☐ d) more superficial blood vessels

21 Which anatomical feature is responsible for fingerprints?

- ☐ a) ridge patterns in the thick skin covering the fingertips
- ☐ b) dermal papillae
- ☐ c) the thickness of stratum lucidum
- ☐ d) the architectural arrangement of melanocytes

Fill-in

Fill in the following blanks in the spaces provided to the right.

22 From superficial to deep, the two layers of the cutaneous membrane are the _____ and the _____ .

23 The _____ layer separates the integument from the fascia around deeper organs.

24 _____ sweat glands are found in the axillae, nipples, and pubic region.

25 The most common form of skin cancer is _____ .

26 A deficiency or absence of _____ production leads to a disorder known as albinism.

22 _____ , _____

23 _____

24 _____

25 _____

26 _____

Short answer

27 In which layer(s) of the epidermis does cell division occur?

_____

_____

_____

28 What is the function of the arrector pili muscles?

_____

_____

_____

29 Explain how hair color can vary from person to person, and over a person's lifetime.

_____

_____

_____

30 What are the risks from having inadequate levels of vitamin D_3 in the body?

_____

_____

_____

31 Explain why when warming your hands by a campfire, your face feels the heat more than your hands.

_____

_____

_____

32 Why is it important for a surgeon to choose an incision pattern according to the cleavage lines of the skin?

_____

_____

_____

33 A 32-year-old woman is admitted to the hospital with third-degree burns on her entire right leg, entire right arm, and the back of her trunk. Estimate the percentage of her surface area that is affected by these burns.

_____

_____

_____

Concept map

Use each of the following terms once to fill in the blank boxes to correctly complete the map.

- lacunae
- osteocytes
- collagen
- intramembranous ossification
- compact bone
- periosteum
- hyaline cartilage

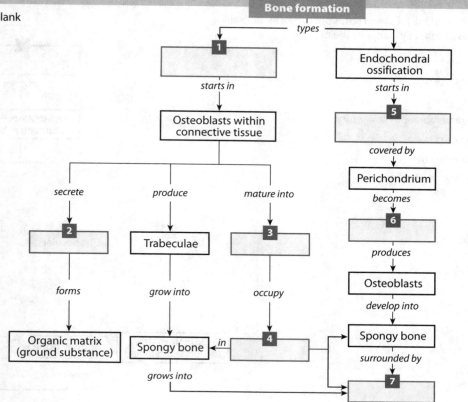

Bone formation

types

1 ☐

Endochondral ossification

starts in → Osteoblasts within connective tissue

starts in → 5 ☐

covered by → Perichondrium

becomes → 6 ☐

produces → Osteoblasts

develop into → Spongy bone

secrete → 2 ☐
produce → Trabeculae
mature into → 3 ☐

forms → Organic matrix (ground substance)

grow into → Spongy bone

occupy → 4 ☐ *in* Spongy bone

grows into

surrounded by → 7 ☐

Vocabulary

Write the term for each of the following descriptions in the space provided.

8 Bones with complex shapes

9 The expanded ends of a long bone

10 A shallow depression in the surface of a bone

11 The marrow-filled space within a bone

12 The strut- and plate-shaped matrix of spongy bone

13 Cells that remove and recycle bone matrix

14 Bones that develop in tendons

15 The process that forms new bone matrix

16 The basic functional unit of compact bone

17 Type of bone growth that increases bone diameter

18 Process by which cartilage is replaced by bone

8 _____

9 _____

10 _____

11 _____

12 _____

13 _____

14 _____

15 _____

16 _____

17 _____

18 _____

Section integration

While playing on her swing set, 10-year-old Rebecca falls and breaks her right leg. At the emergency room, the doctor tells her parents that the proximal end of the tibia where the epiphysis meets the diaphysis is fractured. The fracture is properly set and eventually heals. During a routine physical when she is 18, Rebecca learns that her right leg is 2.54 cm (1 in.) shorter than her left. What might account for this difference?

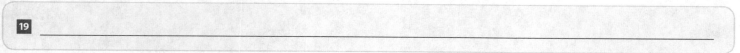

19 _____

51

Concept map

Use each of the following terms once to fill in the blank boxes to correctly complete the map.

- lacunae
- osteocytes
- collagen
- intramembranous ossification
- compact bone
- periosteum
- hyaline cartilage

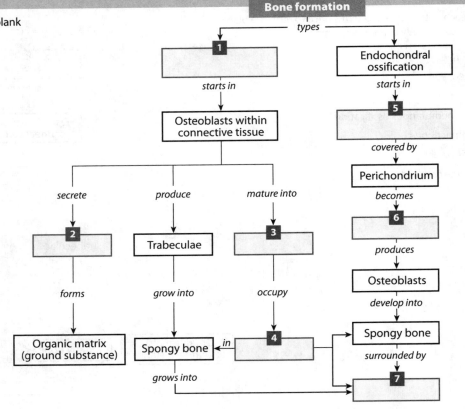

Vocabulary

Write the term for each of the following descriptions in the space provided.

8	Bones with complex shapes
9	The expanded ends of a long bone
10	A shallow depression in the surface of a bone
11	The marrow-filled space within a bone
12	The strut- and plate-shaped matrix of spongy bone
13	Cells that remove and recycle bone matrix
14	Bones that develop in tendons
15	The process that forms new bone matrix
16	The basic functional unit of compact bone
17	Type of bone growth that increases bone diameter
18	Process by which cartilage is replaced by bone

Section integration

While playing on her swing set, 10-year-old Rebecca falls and breaks her right leg. At the emergency room, the doctor tells her parents that the proximal end of the tibia where the epiphysis meets the diaphysis is fractured. The fracture is properly set and eventually heals. During a routine physical when she is 18, Rebecca learns that her right leg is 2.54 cm (1 in.) shorter than her left. What might account for this difference?

19 _____

Concept map

Use each of the following terms once to fill in the blank boxes to correctly complete the map.

- ↓ Ca^{2+} level
- homeostasis
- release of stored Ca^{2+} from bone
- ↓ Ca^{2+} concentration in blood
- parathyroid glands
- calcitonin
- ↑ Ca^{2+} concentration in blood

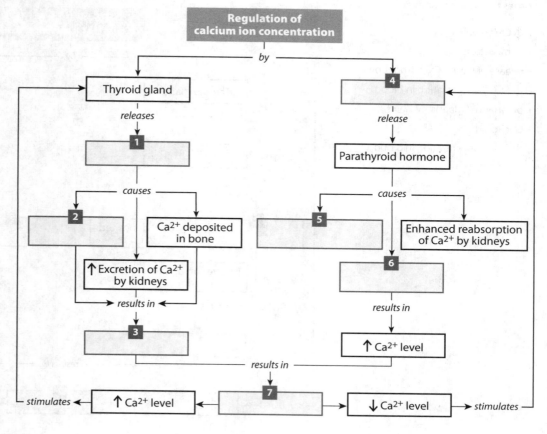

Regulation of calcium ion concentration

by

Thyroid gland — *releases* → [1]

[4] — *release* → Parathyroid hormone

[1] — *causes* → [2] ; Ca²⁺ deposited in bone

[2] → ↑ Excretion of Ca²⁺ by kidneys

results in → [3]

Parathyroid hormone — *causes* → [5] ; Enhanced reabsorption of Ca²⁺ by kidneys

[5] → [6]

results in → ↑ Ca²⁺ level

results in → [7]

stimulates ← ↑ Ca²⁺ level ← [7] → ↓ Ca²⁺ level → *stimulates*

Short answer

Identify the type of fracture and the bones involved in each of the following x-ray images.

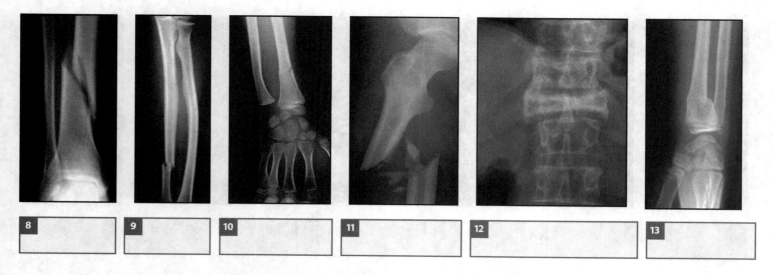

| 8 | 9 | 10 | 11 | 12 | 13 |

Concept map

Use each of the following terms once to fill in the blank boxes to correctly complete the map.

- ↓ Ca^{2+} level
- homeostasis
- release of stored Ca^{2+} from bone
- ↓ Ca^{2+} concentration in blood
- parathyroid glands
- calcitonin
- ↑ Ca^{2+} concentration in blood

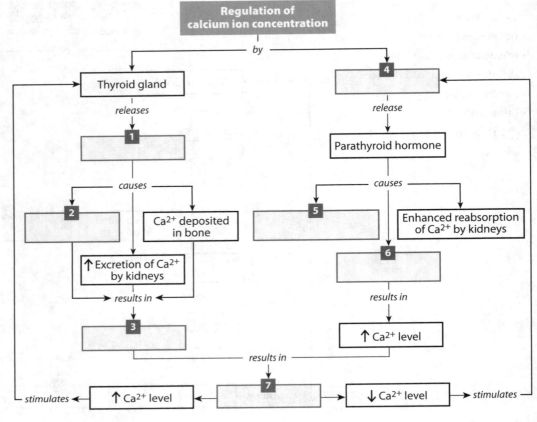

Regulation of calcium ion concentration

by

Thyroid gland

releases

1

causes

2 Ca^{2+} deposited in bone

↑ Excretion of Ca^{2+} by kidneys

results in

3

4

release

Parathyroid hormone

causes

5   Enhanced reabsorption of Ca^{2+} by kidneys

6

results in

↑ Ca^{2+} level

results in

stimulates ← ↑ Ca^{2+} level ← **7** → ↓ Ca^{2+} level → *stimulates*

Short answer

Identify the type of fracture and the bones involved in each of the following x-ray images.

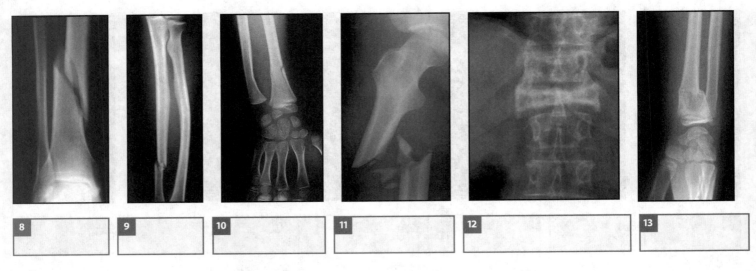

8

9

10

11

12

13

Chapter Review Questions

Labeling

Identify the anatomical regions and structures in this image of a long bone.

| 1 |
| 2 |
| 3 |
| 4 |
| 5 |
| 6 |
| 7 |

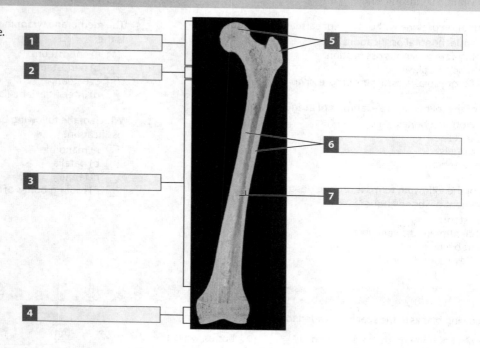

True/False

Indicate whether each statement is true or false.

8 A broken leg that results in a bone protruding through the skin is called a compound fracture.

9 The primary ossification centers are localized in the epiphyses.

10 Osteoblastic activity tends to deposit calcium into the bone.

11 Parathyroid hormone (PTH) is released in response to low blood calcium levels.

12 Cancellous bone and compact bone are synonymous terms.

13 A foramen is a small rounded passageway through which blood vessels or nerves penetrate.

14 Bone has a rich blood supply, but lacks sensory innervation.

15 Appositional growth increases bone diameter.

8 _____

9 _____

10 _____

11 _____

12 _____

13 _____

14 _____

15 _____

Multiple choice

Select the correct answer from the list provided.

16 Blood cell formation occurs in
- a) yellow bone marrow.
- b) red bone marrow.
- c) the matrix of bone tissue.
- d) the ground substance of bones.

17 Which of the following hormones is *not* involved with blood calcium ion homeostasis?
- a) calcitriol
- b) parathyroid hormone
- c) prolactin
- d) calcitonin

18 The presence of an epiphyseal line indicates
- a) epiphyseal growth has ended.
- b) the bone is fractured at that location.
- c) the bone will continue increasing in length for many years.
- d) vitamin D3 insufficiency.

19 The formation of bone without a prior cartilaginous model is
- a) endochondral ossification.
- b) intramembranous ossification.
- c) achondroplasia.
- d) fibrodysplasia ossificans progressiva.

20 Which of the following are examples of irregular bones?
- a) Wormian bones
- b) patellae
- c) carpals
- d) vertebrae

21 Which of the following terms is used to describe the architectural arrangement of spongy bone?
- a) osteon
- b) circumferential lamellae
- c) trabeculae
- d) Haversian system

22 Red bone marrow resides in the
- a) medullary cavity.
- b) sinus cavity.
- c) facets.
- d) fossa.

23 The membrane wrapping the bones, except at the joint cavity, is the
- a) endosteum.
- b) periosteum.
- c) osteon.
- d) interstitial lamellae.

24 Which of the following bones is *not* formed by endochondral ossification?
- a) mandible
- b) patella
- c) femur
- d) roofing bones of the skull

Fill-in

Fill in the following blanks in the spaces provided to the right.

25 The number of bones in the axial skeleton is _____ bones, while the appendicular skeleton contains _____ bones.

26 _____ bones develop inside tendons and are commonly located near the joints of the knees, hands, and feet.

27 An air-filled chamber within a bone is called a(an) _____.

28 The functional unit of mature compact bone is called a(an) _____.

29 _____ are cells that remove and recycle bone matrix.

25 _____ , _____

26 _____

27 _____

28 _____

29 _____

Short answer

30 What are the five primary functions of the skeletal system?

_____

_____

_____

31 Which kind of fracture would you expect to occur in a patient whose shinbone broke when her foot stuck to the floor while she was dancing a pirouette?

_____

_____

_____

32 Compare and contrast pituitary growth failure and achondroplasia.

_____

_____

_____

33 What is the primary difference between endochondral ossification and intramembranous ossification?

_____

_____

_____

34 Describe why epiphyseal fractures are of particular concern.

_____

_____

_____

35 Why are impacts perpendicular to the shaft of a long bone more dangerous than stress applied parallel to the long axis of the bone?

_____

_____

_____

36 Distinguish between acromegaly and gigantism.

_____

_____

_____

Labeling

In the image below, label the bones of the orbital complex.

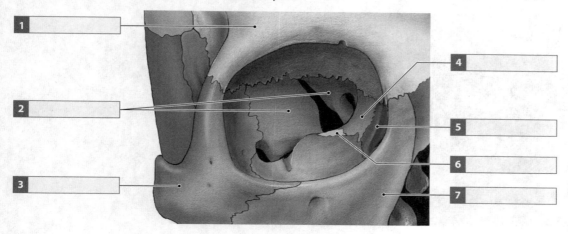

1. _____

2. _____

3. _____

4. _____

5. _____

6. _____

7. _____

In the images below, label the sutures and fontanelles of the infant skull.

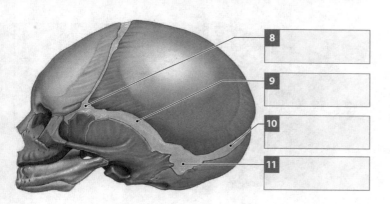

8. _____

9. _____

10. _____

11. _____

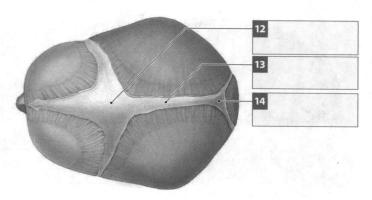

12. _____

13. _____

14. _____

Short answer

Identify the vertebral region and regional characteristics for each vertebra.

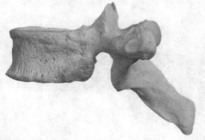

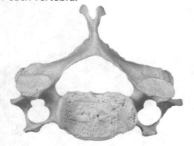

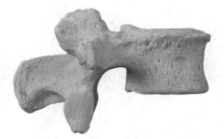

15. Region:

16. Characteristics:

17. Region:

18. Characteristics:

19. Region:

20. Characteristics:

Labeling

In the image below, label the bones of the orbital complex.

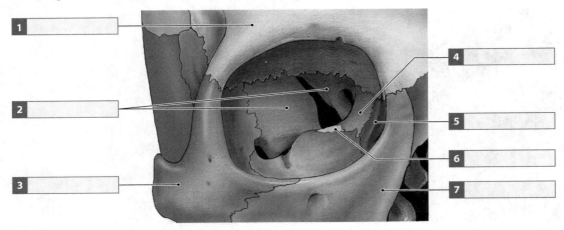

1 [_____]

2 [_____]

3 [_____]

4 [_____]

5 [_____]

6 [_____]

7 [_____]

In the images below, label the sutures and fontanelles of the infant skull.

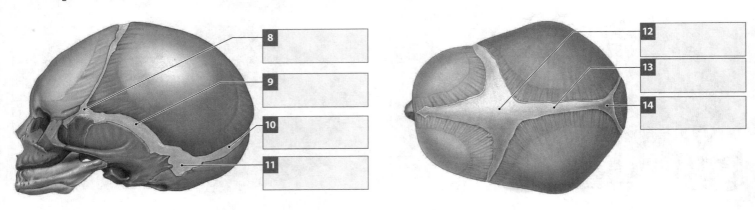

8 [_____]

9 [_____]

10 [_____]

11 [_____]

12 [_____]

13 [_____]

14 [_____]

Short answer

Identify the vertebral region and regional characteristics for each vertebra.

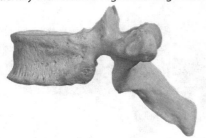

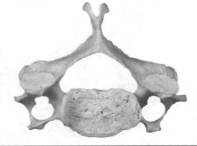

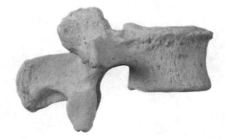

15 Region:

16 Characteristics:

17 Region:

18 Characteristics:

19 Region:

20 Characteristics:

Labeling

Label the bones of the appendicular skeleton in the diagram at right.

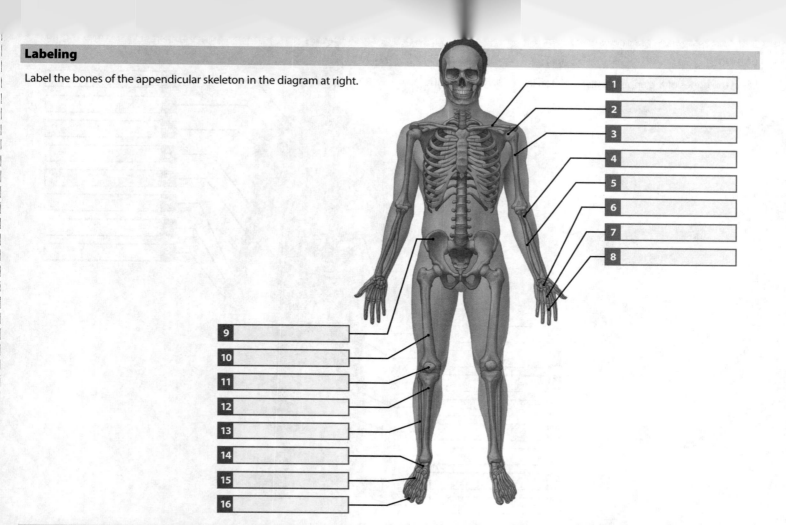

1	
2	
3	
4	
5	
6	
7	
8	

9	
10	
11	
12	
13	
14	
15	
16	

Short answer

In the pelvis diagrams below, identify the sex and the differences between them.

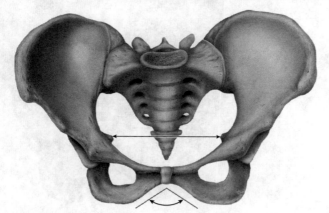

17	Sex:
18	**Differences:**

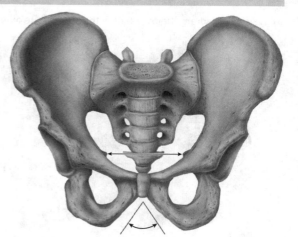

19	Sex:
20	**Differences:**

Labeling

Label the bones of the appendicular skeleton in the diagram at right.

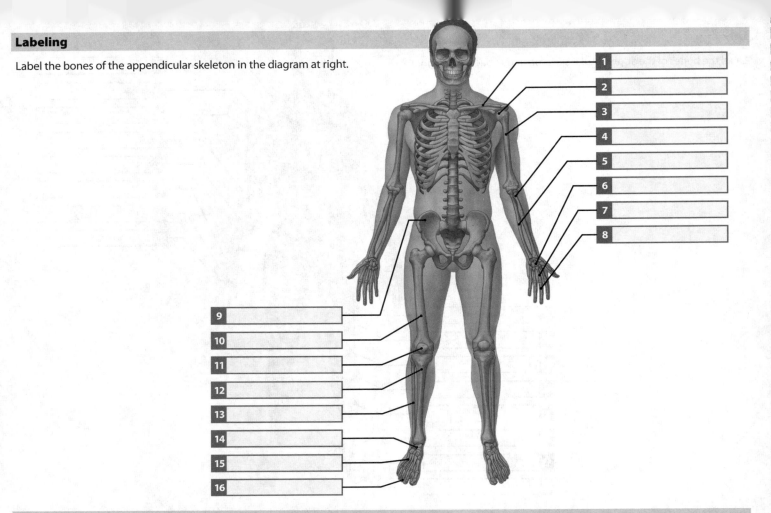

1	
2	
3	
4	
5	
6	
7	
8	

9	
10	
11	
12	
13	
14	
15	
16	

Short answer

In the pelvis diagrams below, identify the sex and the differences between them.

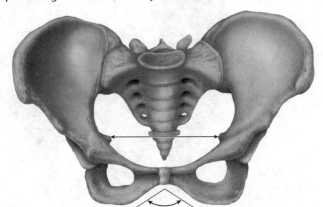

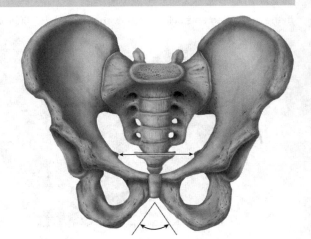

17	Sex:
18	Differences:

19	Sex:
20	Differences:

Chapter Review Questions

Labeling

Identify the cranial and facial bones in the diagrams below.

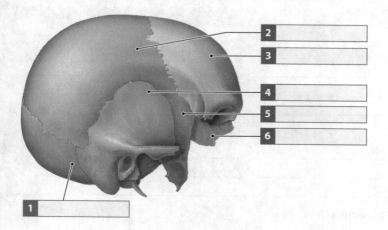

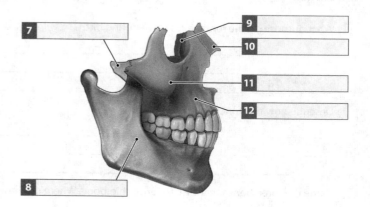

True/False

Indicate whether each statement is true or false.

13　The patella is a sesamoid bone.

14　The adductor tubercle is a small pit in the center of the femoral head.

15　The lateral border of the scapula is also called the vertebral border.

16　The last two pairs of ribs are also called floating ribs.

13 _____

14 _____

15 _____

16 _____

Multiple choice

Select the correct answer from the list provided.

17　When you move your head as if to say no,
- a) the atlas rotates on the occipital condyles.
- b) C_1 and C_2 rotate on the adjoining cervical vertebrae.
- c) the atlas rotates on the dens of the axis.
- d) the skull rotates with both C_1 and C_2.

18　Which of the following pairs of bones make up the bony nasal septum?
- a) inferior nasal conchae and vomer
- b) perpendicular plate of ethmoid and inferior nasal conchae
- c) vomer and perpendicular plate of ethmoid
- d) inferior nasal conchae and middle nasal conchae of ethmoid

19　The unpaired facial bones include the
- a) lacrimal and nasal.
- b) vomer and mandible.
- c) maxilla and mandible.
- d) zygomatic and palatine.

20　The joint between the frontal and parietal bones is correctly called the
- a) parietal suture.
- b) lambdoid suture.
- c) squamous suture.
- d) coronal suture.

21　Which part of the ulna forms the point of the elbow?
- a) styloid process
- b) olecranon
- c) coronoid process
- d) trochlear notch

22　Which of the following bones is *not* part of the orbital complex?
- a) lacrimal
- b) nasal
- c) ethmoid
- d) sphenoid

23 The head of the femur articulates with the pelvis at the
- [ ] a) true pelvis.
- [ ] b) acetabulum.
- [ ] c) obturator foramen.
- [ ] d) pubic symphysis.

24 What is the name of the flexible sheet that interconnects the radius and ulna (and the tibia and fibula)?
- [ ] a) interosseous membrane
- [ ] b) obturator foramen
- [ ] c) linea aspera
- [ ] d) intercondylar eminence

Short answer

25 What purpose do the fontanelles serve during birth?

_____

_____

_____

26 Describe how ribs function in breathing.

_____

_____

_____

27 Name the three bones that fuse to form a hip bone. Where do these bones meet?

_____

_____

_____

28 Distinguish between the primary and secondary curves of the vertebral column.

_____

_____

_____

29 Describe the arches of the feet.

_____

_____

_____

Labeling

Label the structures in the synovial joint figure at right.

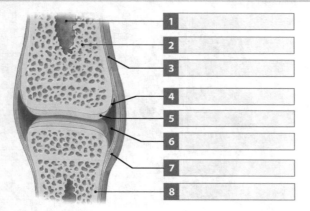

1 _____
2 _____
3 _____
4 _____
5 _____
6 _____
7 _____
8 _____

Identify each of the following movements.

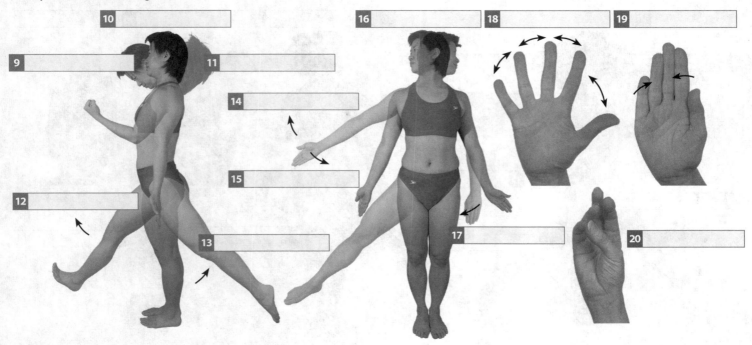

9 _____
10 _____
11 _____
12 _____
13 _____
14 _____
15 _____
16 _____
17 _____
18 _____
19 _____
20 _____

Matching

Match each lettered term with the most closely related description.

a. amphiarthrosis
b. synarthrosis
c. dislocation
d. pronation/supination
e. diarthrosis
f. shoulder
g. articular discs
h. fluid-filled pouch

21 Freely movable joint
22 Movements of forearm bones
23 Ball-and-socket joint
24 Menisci
25 Immovable joint
26 Luxation
27 Bursa
28 Slightly movable joint

21 _____
22 _____
23 _____
24 _____
25 _____
26 _____
27 _____
28 _____

65

Labeling

Label the structures in the synovial joint figure at right.

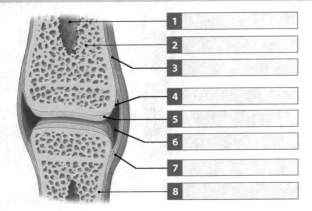

1 _____

2 _____

3 _____

4 _____

5 _____

6 _____

7 _____

8 _____

Identify each of the following movements.

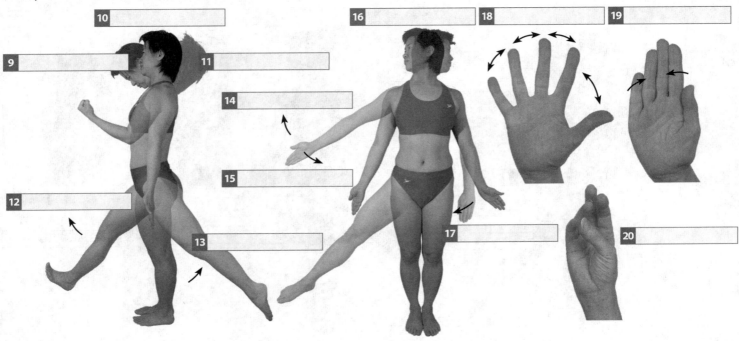

9 _____

10 _____

11 _____

12 _____

13 _____

14 _____

15 _____

16 _____

17 _____

18 _____

19 _____

20 _____

Matching

Match each lettered term with the most closely related description.

a. amphiarthrosis

b. synarthrosis

c. dislocation

d. pronation/supination

e diarthrosis

f. shoulder

g. articular discs

h. fluid-filled pouch

21 Freely movable joint

22 Movements of forearm bones

23 Ball-and-socket joint

24 Menisci

25 Immovable joint

26 Luxation

27 Bursa

28 Slightly movable joint

21 _____

22 _____

23 _____

24 _____

25 _____

26 _____

27 _____

28 _____

Labeling

Label each of the structures in the accompanying diagram of the shoulder joint.

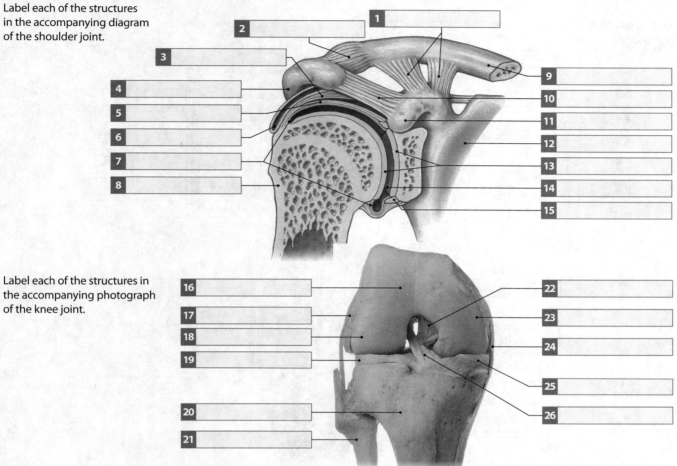

1
2
3
4
5
6
7
8
9
10
11
12
13
14
15

Label each of the structures in the accompanying photograph of the knee joint.

16
17
18
19
20
21
22
23
24
25
26

Matching

Match each lettered term with the most closely related description.

a. acetabulum
b. popliteal ligament
c. disc outer layer
d. dislocation
e. arthritis
f. disc inner layer
g. reinforce knee joint
h. osteoporosis

27 Knee joint posterior
28 Articular cartilage damage
29 Reduced bone mass
30 Cruciate ligaments
31 Anulus fibrosus
32 Deep fossa
33 Nucleus pulposus
34 Nursemaid's elbow

27 _____
28 _____
29 _____
30 _____
31 _____
32 _____
33 _____
34 _____

Short answer

35 Identify the joints that attach the pectoral and pelvic girdles to the axial skeleton.

_____
_____

Labeling

Label each of the structures in the accompanying diagram of the shoulder joint.

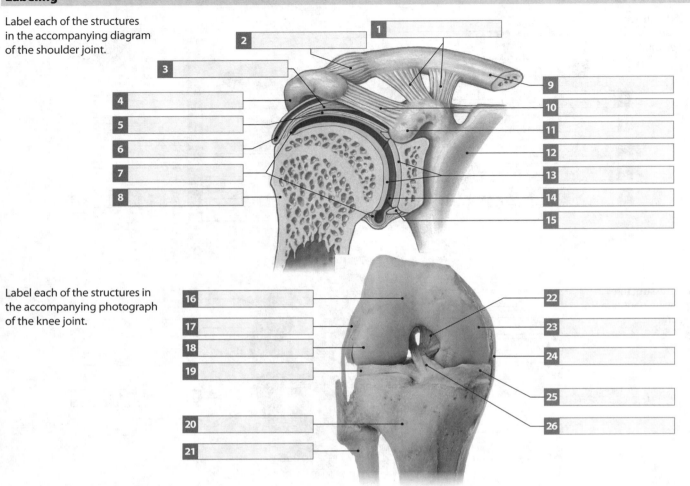

1	
2	
3	
4	
5	
6	
7	
8	
9	
10	
11	
12	
13	
14	
15	

Label each of the structures in the accompanying photograph of the knee joint.

16	
17	
18	
19	
20	
21	
22	
23	
24	
25	
26	

Matching

Match each lettered term with the most closely related description.

a. acetabulum
b. popliteal ligament
c. disc outer layer
d. dislocation
e. arthritis
f. disc inner layer
g. reinforce knee joint
h. osteoporosis

27 Knee joint posterior
28 Articular cartilage damage
29 Reduced bone mass
30 Cruciate ligaments
31 Anulus fibrosus
32 Deep fossa
33 Nucleus pulposus
34 Nursemaid's elbow

27 _____
28 _____
29 _____
30 _____
31 _____
32 _____
33 _____
34 _____

Short answer

35 Identify the joints that attach the pectoral and pelvic girdles to the axial skeleton.

_____
_____

Chapter Review Questions

True/False

Indicate whether each statement is true or false.

1 A bursa is a synovial fluid pocket outside of a joint capsule.

2 The acromioclavicular joint is an example of a condylar joint.

3 Standing up from a chair involves hip joint extension and knee joint flexion.

4 The ligamentum flavum connects the laminae of adjacent vertebrae.

5 The nucleus pulposus provides resiliency and shock absorption to the intervertebral disc.

6 The ligamentum teres attaches the head of the humerus into the glenoid cavity.

1	_____
2	_____
3	_____
4	_____
5	_____
6	_____

Multiple choice

Select the correct answer from the list provided.

7 The synarthrosis formed between the bones of the skull is a
- ☐ a) gomphosis.
- ☐ b) synostosis.
- ☐ c) symphysis.
- ☐ d) suture.

8 The joint between adjacent vertebral bodies is a
- ☐ a) synostosis.
- ☐ b) syndesmosis.
- ☐ c) symphysis.
- ☐ d) gomphosis.

9 The joints typically located at the end of adjacent long bones are
- ☐ a) synarthroses.
- ☐ b) amphiarthroses.
- ☐ c) diarthroses.
- ☐ d) symphyses.

10 The function of articular cartilage is to
- ☐ a) reduce friction.
- ☐ b) prevent bony surfaces from contacting one another.
- ☐ c) provide lubrication.
- ☐ d) both a and b

11 Which of the following is *not* a function of synovial fluid?
- ☐ a) shock absorption
- ☐ b) nutrient distribution
- ☐ c) lubrication of articular surfaces
- ☐ d) maintenance of ionic balance

12 A dislocation of an articulating surface is
- ☐ a) circumduction.
- ☐ b) hyperextension.
- ☐ c) luxation.
- ☐ d) supination.

13 Abduction and adduction always refer to movements of the
- ☐ a) axial skeleton.
- ☐ b) appendicular skeleton.
- ☐ c) skull.
- ☐ d) vertebral column.

14 Rotation of the radius that makes the palm face posteriorly is
- ☐ a) supination.
- ☐ b) pronation.
- ☐ c) protraction.
- ☐ d) inversion.

15 A ballerina standing on her toes is performing which action of the ankle joint?
- ☐ a) dorsiflexion
- ☐ b) plantar flexion
- ☐ c) inversion
- ☐ d) eversion

16 Increasing the angle between bones is
- ☐ a) flexion.
- ☐ b) extension.
- ☐ c) hyperextension.
- ☐ d) abduction.

17 The hip is an extremely stable joint because it has

- ☐ a) a complete bony socket.
- ☐ b) a strong articular capsule.
- ☐ c) supporting ligaments.
- ☐ d) all of the above

18 Movement of a limb away from the longitudinal axis of the body is

- ☐ a) abduction.
- ☐ b) adduction.
- ☐ c) hyperextension.
- ☐ d) protraction.

19 Although the knee is only considered to be one joint, how many separate joints does it actually contain?

- ☐ a) two
- ☐ b) three
- ☐ c) four
- ☐ d) five

20 The head of the radius is attached to the ulna by the

- ☐ a) radial collateral ligament.
- ☐ b) ulnar collateral ligament.
- ☐ c) annular ligament.
- ☐ d) medial cruciate ligament.

Short answer

21 Differentiate between a bulging disc and a herniated disc.

_____
_____
_____

22 Explain how articular cartilage differs from other cartilage in the body.

_____
_____
_____

23 List the six different types of diarthroses, and give an example of each.

_____
_____
_____

24 Describe how a meniscus functions in a joint.

_____
_____
_____

25 Distinguish between osteopenia and osteoporosis.

_____
_____
_____

Labeling

Label the structures in this figure of a skeletal muscle fiber.

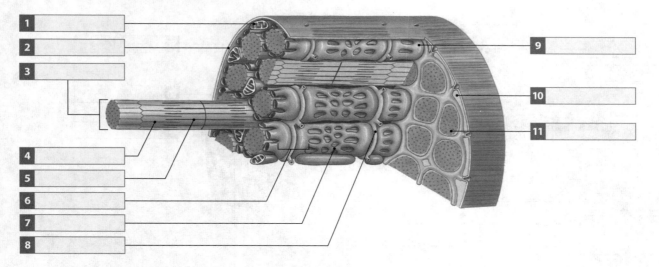

1 _____
2 _____
3 _____

9 _____

10 _____

11 _____

4 _____
5 _____
6 _____
7 _____
8 _____

Label the structures in this diagram of adjacent sarcomeres.

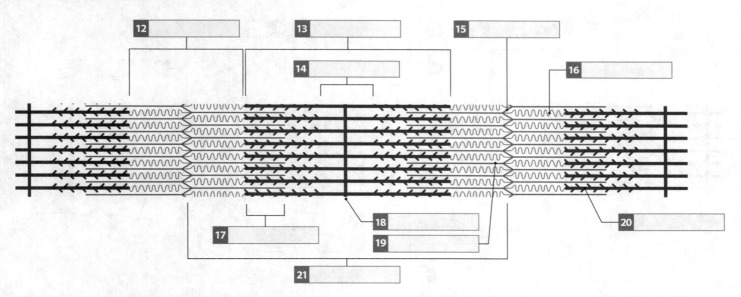

12 _____

13 _____

15 _____

14 _____

16 _____

17 _____

18 _____

19 _____

20 _____

21 _____

Fill-in

In the spaces provided, reorder the following terms in their proper sequence from largest (22) to smallest (27).

- muscle fiber
- muscle fascicle
- sarcomere
- myofibril
- skeletal muscle
- myofilament

22 _____

23 _____

24 _____

25 _____

26 _____

27 _____

Labeling

Label the structures in this figure of a skeletal muscle fiber.

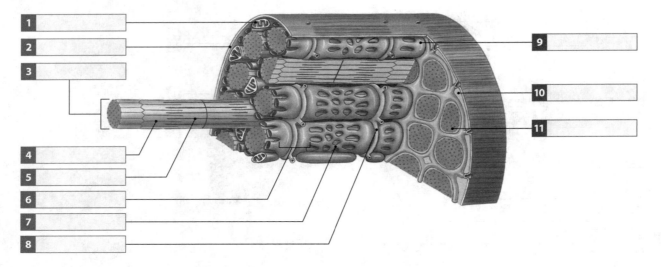

1. _____
2. _____
3. _____

4. _____
5. _____
6. _____
7. _____
8. _____

9. _____
10. _____
11. _____

Label the structures in this diagram of adjacent sarcomeres.

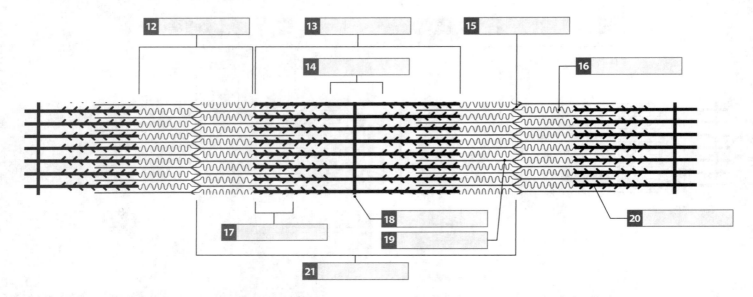

12. _____
13. _____
14. _____
15. _____
16. _____

17. _____
18. _____
19. _____
20. _____
21. _____

Fill-in

In the spaces provided, reorder the following terms in their proper sequence from largest (22) to smallest (27).

- muscle fiber
- muscle fascicle
- sarcomere
- myofibril
- skeletal muscle
- myofilament

22. _____
23. _____
24. _____
25. _____
26. _____
27. _____

Labeling

Use the following terms to correctly label the structures in the diagram representing a blood vessel and a skeletal muscle at rest.

- creatine
- glycogen
- CP
- glucose
- O_2
- fatty acids

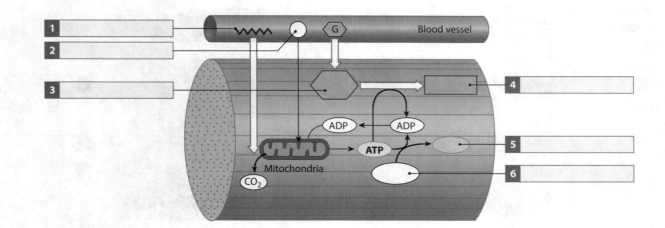

Matching

Match each lettered term with the most closely related description.

a. eccentric contraction

b. isometric contraction

c. isotonic contraction

d. concentric contraction

7 Muscle does not change length during contraction

8 Muscle changes length during contraction

9 Peak tension less than load, and muscle elongates

10 Peak tension greater than load, and muscle shortens

7 _____

8 _____

9 _____

10 _____

Short answer

Complete the following table by writing in the anatomical and physiological properties of the three types of skeletal muscle fibers.

Property	Fast Fibers	Slow Fibers	Intermediate Fibers
Cross-sectional diameter	**11**	**12**	**13**
Color	**14**	*RED*	**15**
Myoglobin content	**16**	**17**	*LOW*
Capillary supply	*SCARCE*	**18**	**19**
Mitochondria	**20**	**21**	**22**
Time to peak tension	**23**	*PROLONGED*	**24**
Contraction speed	**25**	**26**	**27**
Fatigue resistance	**28**	**29**	*INTERMEDIATE*
Glycolytic enzyme concentration in cytosol	*HIGH*	**30**	**31**

Labeling

Use the following terms to correctly label the structures in the diagram representing a blood vessel and a skeletal muscle at rest.

- creatine
- glycogen
- CP
- glucose
- O_2
- fatty acids

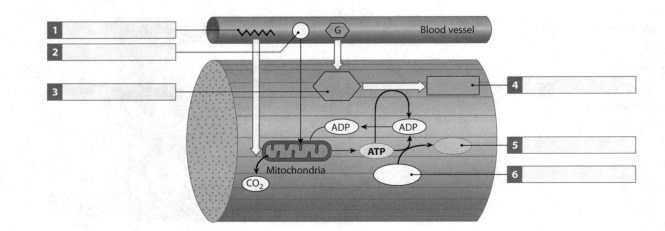

Matching

Match each lettered term with the most closely related description.

a. eccentric contraction

b. isometric contraction

c. isotonic contraction

d. concentric contraction

7	Muscle does not change length during contraction
8	Muscle changes length during contraction
9	Peak tension less than load, and muscle elongates
10	Peak tension greater than load, and muscle shortens

7 _____

8 _____

9 _____

10 _____

Short answer

Complete the following table by writing in the anatomical and physiological properties of the three types of skeletal muscle fibers.

Property	Fast Fibers	Slow Fibers	Intermediate Fibers
Cross-sectional diameter	11	12	13
Color	14	RED	15
Myoglobin content	16	17	LOW
Capillary supply	SCARCE	18	19
Mitochondria	20	21	22
Time to peak tension	23	PROLONGED	24
Contraction speed	25	26	27
Fatigue resistance	28	29	INTERMEDIATE
Glycolytic enzyme concentration in cytosol	HIGH	30	31

Chapter Review Questions

True/False

Indicate whether each statement is true or false.

1 An increase in sarcomere length reduces the tension produced in a muscle fiber by reducing the size of the zone of overlap and the number of potential cross-bridge interactions.

2 Muscle hypertrophy is mostly explained by an increase in muscle fiber (cell) number as a result of exercise.

3 The Cori cycle describes the transfer of lactate to the liver and glucose back to the muscle cells during the recovery period.

4 In glycolysis, one molecule of glucose produces two molecules of pyruvate and 17 ATP.

1 _____

2 _____

3 _____

4 _____

Matching

Match each lettered term with the most closely related description.

a. myoblasts

b. sarcoplasmic reticulum

c. T tubules

d. tropomyosin

e. troponin

f. I band

g. A band

h. synaptic vesicles

i. motor end plate

j. triad

5 Contains Ca^{2+}

6 Contains thick filaments and thin filaments

7 Contain ACh receptors

8 Extensions of the sarcolemma into the sarcoplasm

9 Embryonic cells that fuse to form muscle fibers

10 Contains the neurotransmitter ACh

11 Formed by T tubules and a pair of terminal cisternae

12 Contains only thin filaments

13 Has receptor sites for Ca^{2+}

14 Cover the active sites of the G-actin

5 _____

6 _____

7 _____

8 _____

9 _____

10 _____

11 _____

12 _____

13 _____

14 _____

Multiple choice

Select the correct answer from the list provided.

15 The connective tissue coverings of a skeletal muscle, listed from superficial to deep, are
- a) endomysium, perimysium, and epimysium.
- b) endomysium, epimysium, and perimysium.
- c) epimysium endomysium, and perimysium.
- d) epimysium, perimysium, and endomysium.

16 The detachment of the myosin cross-bridges is directly triggered by
- a) the repolarization of T tubules.
- b) the attachment of ATP to the myosin heads.
- c) the hydrolysis of ATP.
- d) calcium ions.

17 A muscle producing almost peak tension during rapid cycles of contraction and relaxation is said to be in
- a) incomplete tetanus.
- b) treppe.
- c) complete tetanus.
- d) a twitch.

18 The type of contraction in which the tension rises, but the muscle does not change length is
- a) an isotonic contraction.
- b) an isometric contraction.
- c) a concentric contraction.
- d) an eccentric contraction.

19 Which of the following statements about myofibrils is *not* correct?
- a) Each skeletal muscle fiber contains hundreds to thousands of myofibrils.
- b) Myofibrils contain repeating units called sarcomeres.
- c) Myofibrils extend the length of a skeletal muscle fiber.
- d) Filaments consist of bundles of myofibrils.

20 Vesicles filled with acetylcholine (ACh) are found in the
- [ ] a) axon terminal.
- [ ] b) motor end plate.
- [ ] c) synaptic cleft.
- [ ] d) transverse tubule.

21 The properties of slow fibers include all of the following except
- [ ] a) red in color.
- [ ] b) low myoglobin content.
- [ ] c) many mitochondria.
- [ ] d) small cross-sectional diameter.

22 Which of the following activities involves eccentric muscle contractions?
- [ ] a) maintaining upright posture
- [ ] b) lifting a barbell over your head
- [ ] c) lowering yourself into a chair
- [ ] d) blinking your eyes

23 All the muscle fibers controlled by a single motor neuron constitute a
- [ ] a) motor unit.
- [ ] b) motor end plate.
- [ ] c) neuromuscular junction.
- [ ] d) cross-bridge.

24 The region of the A band in a sarcomere that contains only thick filaments is the
- [ ] a) Z line.
- [ ] b) I band.
- [ ] c) zone of overlap.
- [ ] d) H band.

Short answer

25 What structural feature of a skeletal muscle fiber is responsible for conducting action potentials into the interior of the cell?

_____
_____
_____

26 Describe how it is possible that the muscles flexing the elbow can adjust their tension to lift a cup of coffee to your mouth or curl a dumbbell in the gym.

_____
_____
_____

27 Research in exercise physiology suggests that for several days after a bout of intense aerobic exercise, people consume oxygen at a rate greater than when they are normally at rest. Explain these results, and cite the process involved.

_____
_____
_____

28 What two mechanisms are used to generate ATP from glucose in muscle cells?

_____
_____
_____

29 Explain the processes that cause a muscle to hypertrophy.

_____
_____
_____

Labeling

Label each of the muscle types below according to its fascicle organization.

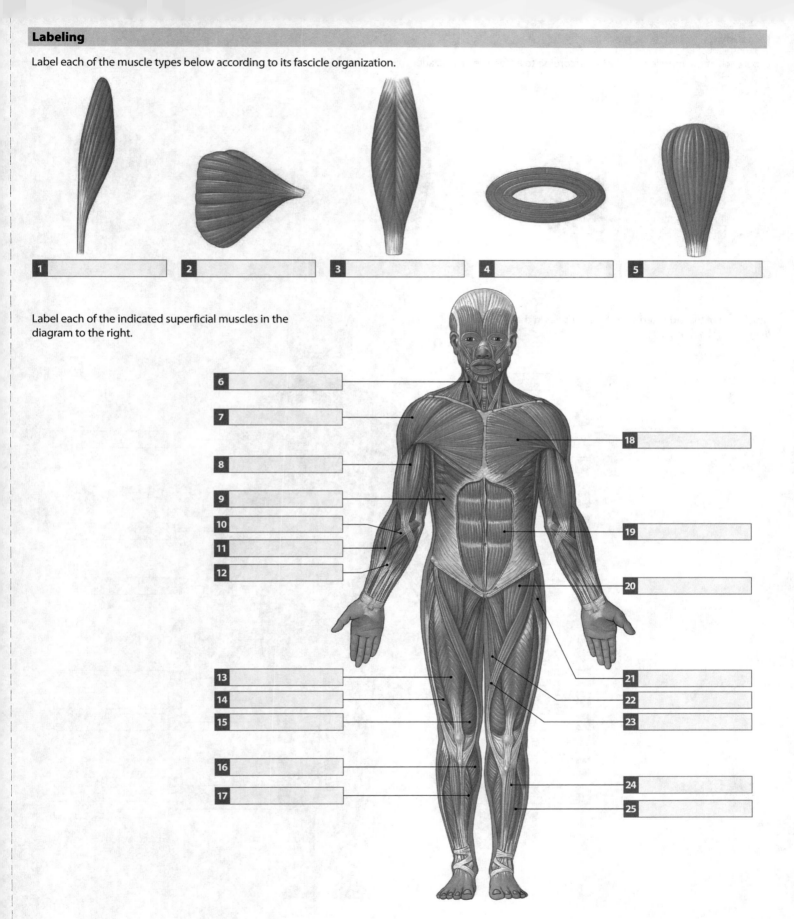

1 [_____]
2 [_____]
3 [_____]
4 [_____]
5 [_____]

Label each of the indicated superficial muscles in the diagram to the right.

6 [_____]
7 [_____]
8 [_____]
9 [_____]
10 [_____]
11 [_____]
12 [_____]
13 [_____]
14 [_____]
15 [_____]
16 [_____]
17 [_____]

18 [_____]
19 [_____]
20 [_____]
21 [_____]
22 [_____]
23 [_____]
24 [_____]
25 [_____]

Labeling

Label each of the muscle types below according to its fascicle organization.

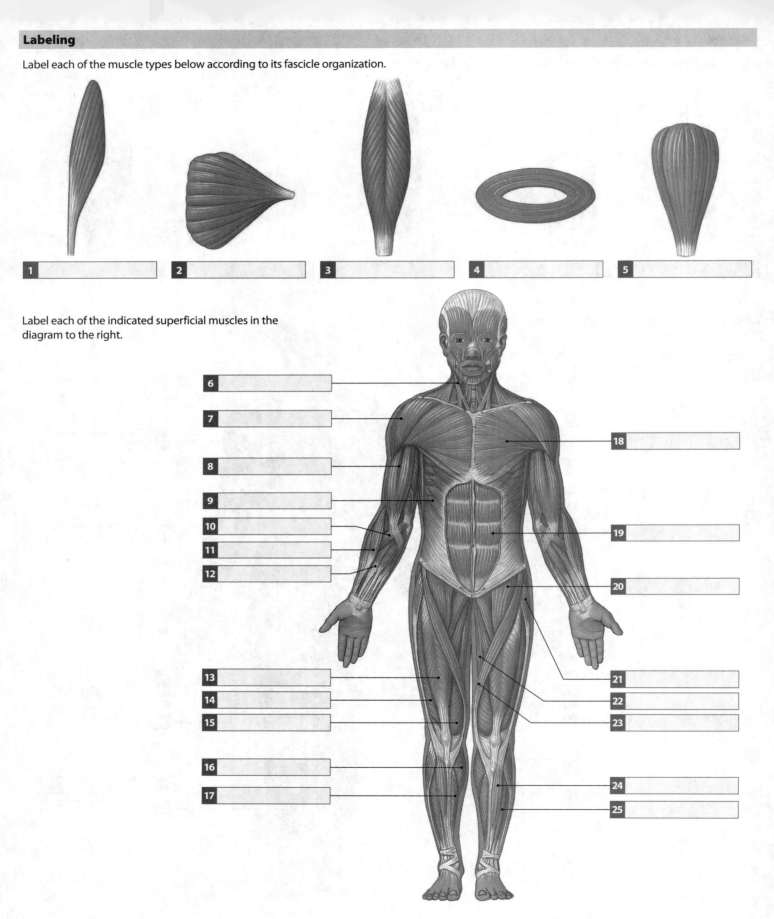

1	
2	
3	
4	
5	

Label each of the indicated superficial muscles in the diagram to the right.

6	
7	
8	
9	
10	
11	
12	
13	
14	
15	
16	
17	

18	
19	
20	
21	
22	
23	
24	
25	

Labeling

Label each of the indicated muscles of the face in the following diagram.

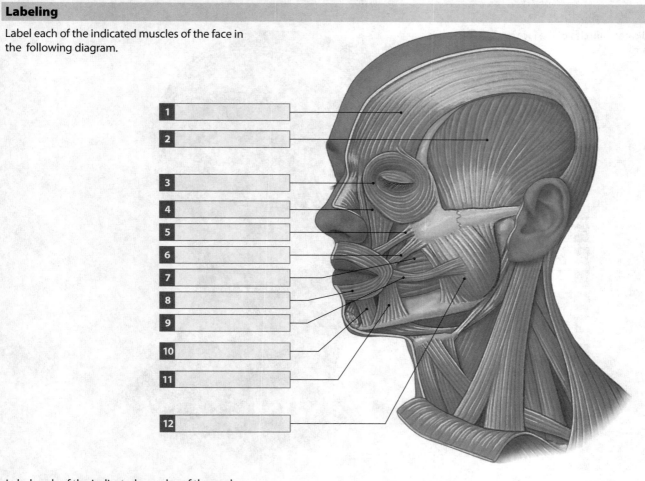

1
2
3
4
5
6
7
8
9
10
11
12

Label each of the indicated muscles of the neck in the following diagram.

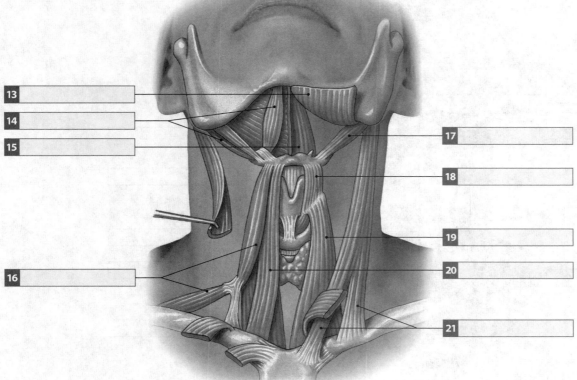

13
14
15
16
17
18
19
20
21

Labeling

Label each of the indicated muscles of the face in the following diagram.

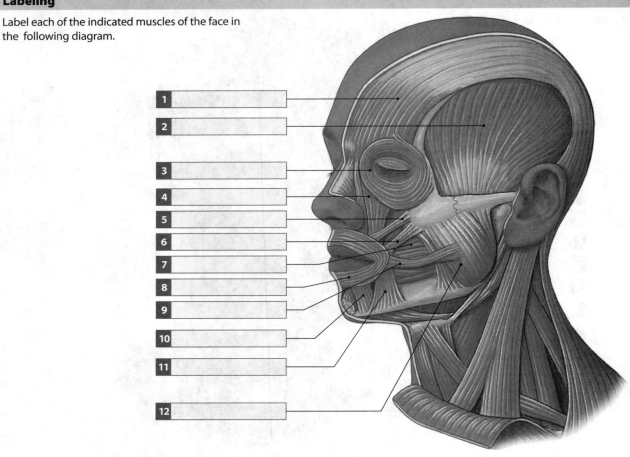

1	
2	
3	
4	
5	
6	
7	
8	
9	
10	
11	
12	

Label each of the indicated muscles of the neck in the following diagram.

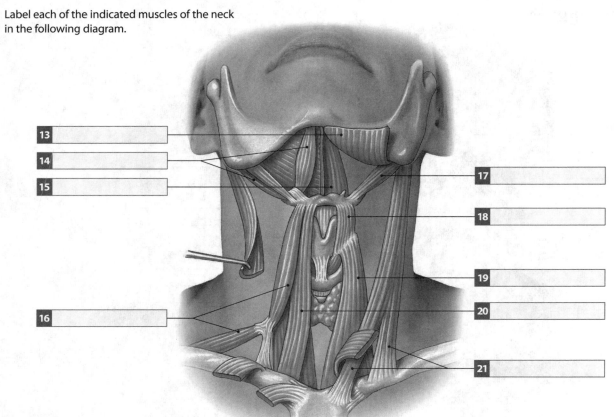

13	
14	
15	
16	
17	
18	
19	
20	
21	

Labeling

Label each of the indicated muscles that move the
forearm and hand in the diagram at right.

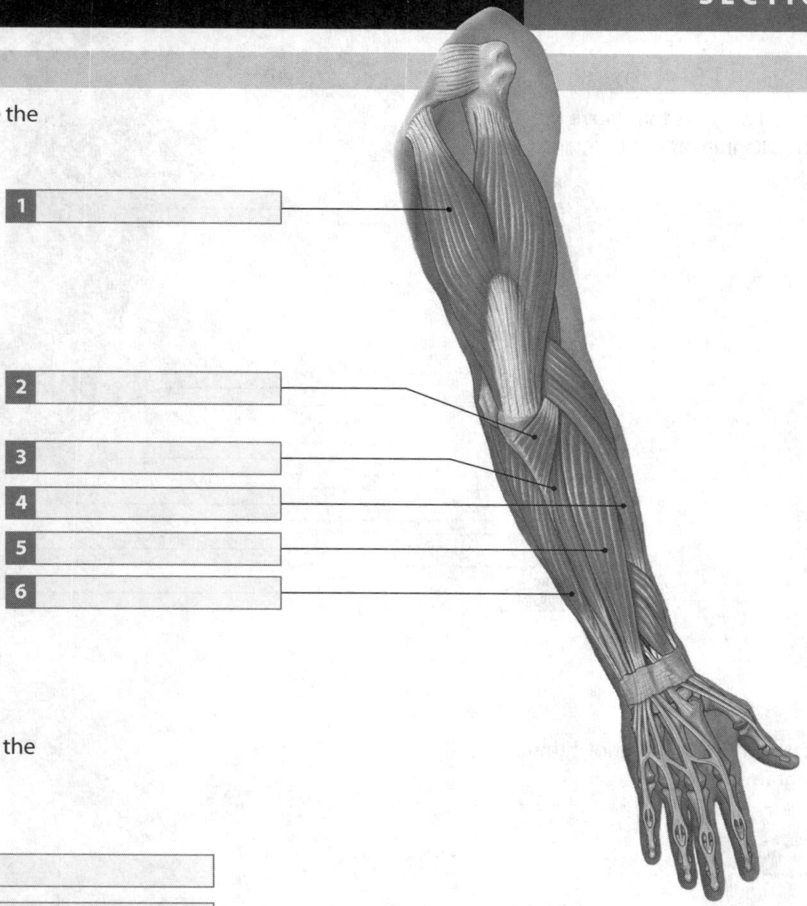

1
2
3
4
5
6

Label each of the indicated muscles that move the
thigh and leg in the diagram below.

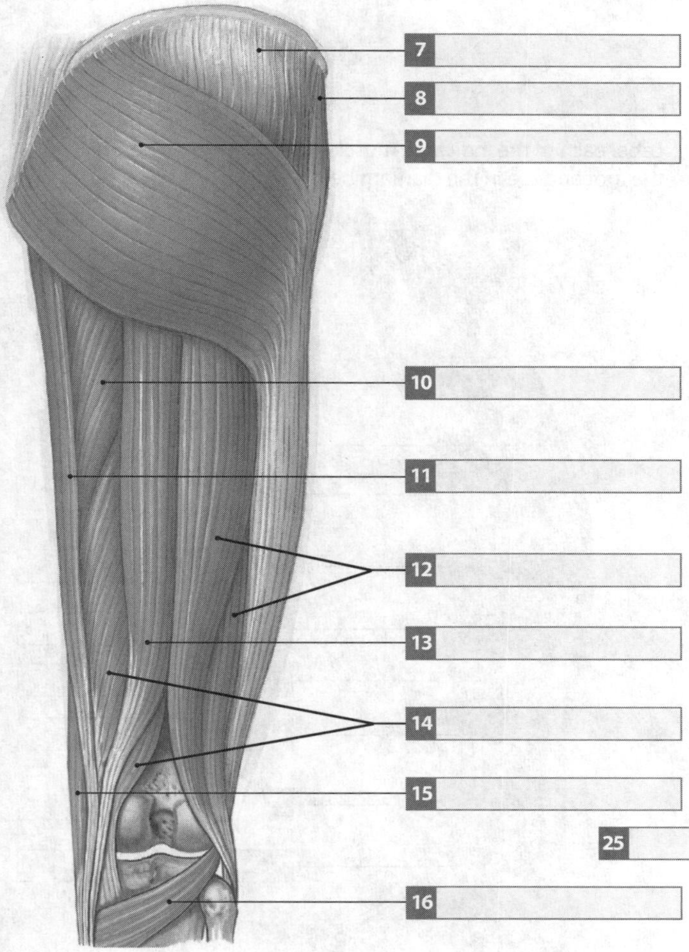

7
8
9

10
11
12
13
14
15
16

Label each of the indicated muscles that move
the foot and toe in the diagram below.

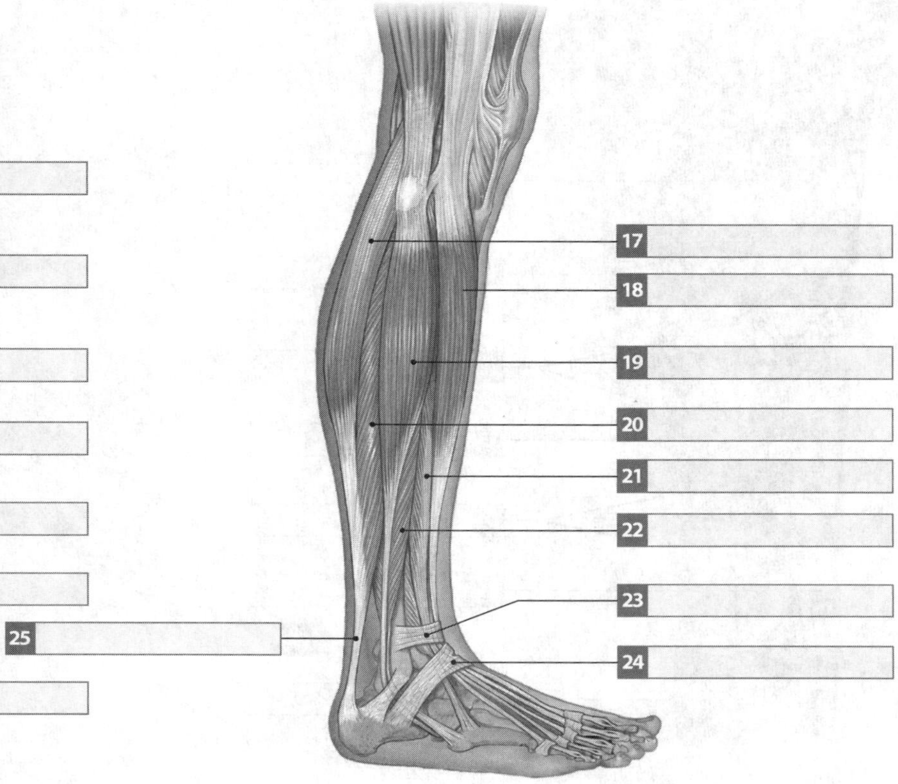

17
18
19
20
21
22
23
24
25

Labeling

Label each of the indicated muscles that move the forearm and hand in the diagram at right.

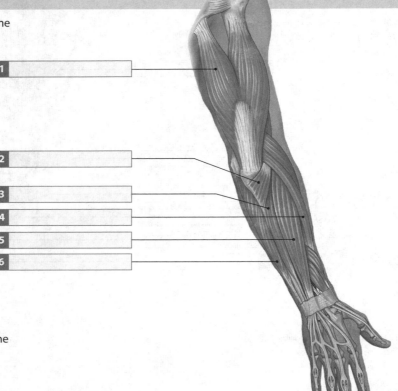

1	
2	
3	
4	
5	
6	

Label each of the indicated muscles that move the thigh and leg in the diagram below.

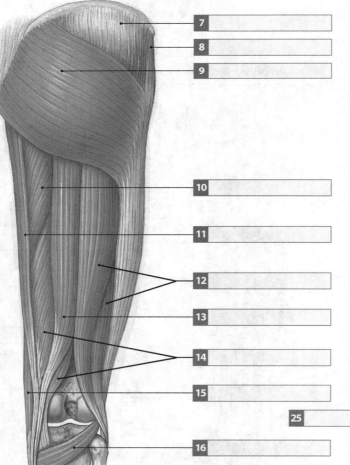

7	
8	
9	
10	
11	
12	
13	
14	
15	
25	
16	

Label each of the indicated muscles that move the foot and toe in the diagram below.

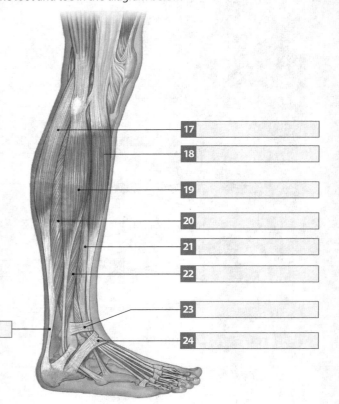

17	
18	
19	
20	
21	
22	
23	
24	

Chapter Review Questions

Labeling

Identify the lever system in each of the images below.

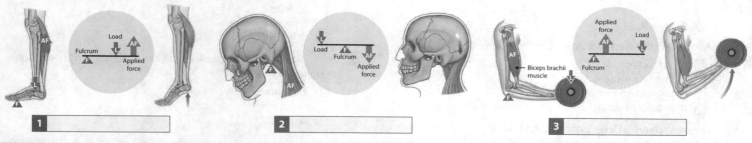

1. _____
2. _____
3. _____

True/False

Indicate whether each statement is true or false.

4. Pectoralis major is an example of a convergent muscle.

5. A wheelbarrow is an example of a third-class lever.

6. A muscle agonist can also be referred to as a prime mover.

7. The inferior rectus and superior oblique are examples of extrinsic eye muscles.

8. The esophageal hiatus is an opening in the transversus abdominis muscle.

4. _____
5. _____
6. _____
7. _____
8. _____

Matching

Match each lettered description with the most closely related muscle.

a. moves eye laterally
b. flexion at knee
c. extension at knee
d. abduction at shoulder
e. downward rotation of scapula
f. flexion at elbow
g. plantar flexion
h. mastication
i. medial rotation at shoulder
j. dorsiflexion

9. Tibialis anterior
10. Temporalis
11. Brachialis
12. Lateral rectus
13. Soleus
14. Biceps femoris
15. Rhomboid major
16. Vastus medialis
17. Deltoid
18. Subscapularis

9. _____
10. _____
11. _____
12. _____
13. _____
14. _____
15. _____
16. _____
17. _____
18. _____

Multiple choice

Select the correct answer from the list provided.

19 The site where the more movable end of a muscle attaches is the
- ☐ a) origin.
- ☐ b) insertion.
- ☐ c) belly.
- ☐ d) fascicle.

20 A muscle with a feather-shaped fascicle organization is called a
- ☐ a) parallel muscle.
- ☐ b) pennate muscle.
- ☐ c) convergent muscle.
- ☐ d) circular muscle.

21 The most common lever system in the body is
- ☐ a) first-class.
- ☐ b) second-class.
- ☐ c) third-class.
- ☐ d) fourth-class.

22 Which of the following muscles is an axial muscle?
- ☐ a) erector spinae
- ☐ b) trapezius
- ☐ c) deltoid
- ☐ d) flexor carpi radialis

23 The major extensor of the elbow is
- ☐ a) triceps brachii.
- ☐ b) biceps brachii.
- ☐ c) deltoid.
- ☐ d) subscapularis.

24 Inflammation of the retinaculum and synovial tendon sheaths resulting in pressure on the median nerve is called
- ☐ a) anterior compartment syndrome.
- ☐ b) rotator cuff syndrome.
- ☐ c) carpal tunnel syndrome.
- ☐ d) plantar fascitis.

25 When doing a pull-up exercise, which of the following muscles is responsible for adduction at the shoulder joint?
- ☐ a) levator scapulae
- ☐ b) deltoid
- ☐ c) supraspinatus
- ☐ d) latissimus dorsi

26 Which of the following muscles performs the hip and knee action required to kick a ball?
- ☐ a) rectus femoris
- ☐ b) pectineus
- ☐ c) gracilis
- ☐ d) biceps femoris

27 Which of the following locations is *not* an attachment site for biceps brachii?
- ☐ a) tuberosity of radius
- ☐ b) coracoid process of scapula
- ☐ c) acromion process of scapula
- ☐ d) supraglenoid tubercle of scapula

28 Which of the following is *not* a muscle of mastication?
- ☐ a) masseter
- ☐ b) buccinator
- ☐ c) temporalis
- ☐ d) lateral pterygoid

Short answer

29 What are the functions of the muscles of the pelvic floor?

_____

_____

_____

30 Identify the muscles of the rotator cuff.

_____

_____

_____

31 List the muscles of the quadriceps muscle group and describe their actions.

_____

_____

_____

_____

Labeling

Label each of the structures in the following diagram of a neuron.

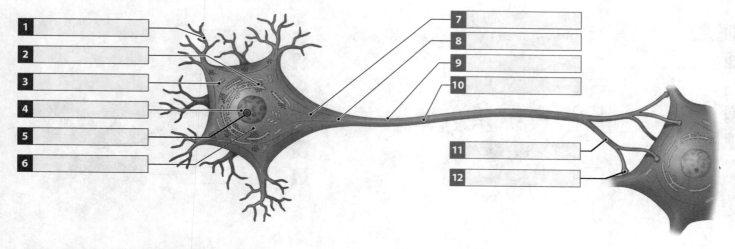

1
2
3
4
5
6

7
8
9
10
11
12

Label the anatomical classes of neurons shown below.

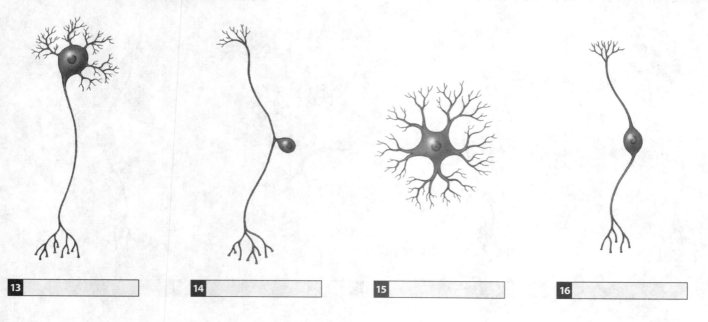

13
14
15
16

Vocabulary

In the space provided, write the boldfaced terms introduced in this section that contain the indicated word part.

17 neur- *(nerve)*   17 _____

18 dendr- *(tree)*   18 _____

19 ef- *(away from)*   19 _____

20 af- *(toward)*   20 _____

Labeling

Label each of the structures in the following diagram of a neuron.

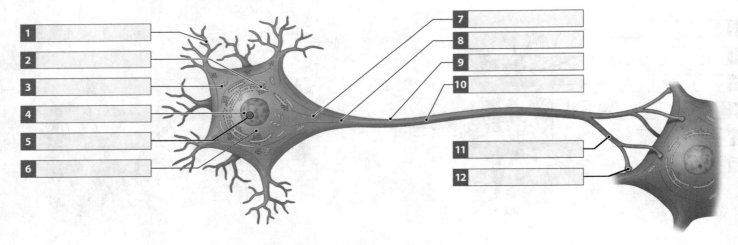

1			7	
2			8	
3			9	
4			10	
5			11	
6			12	

Label the anatomical classes of neurons shown below.

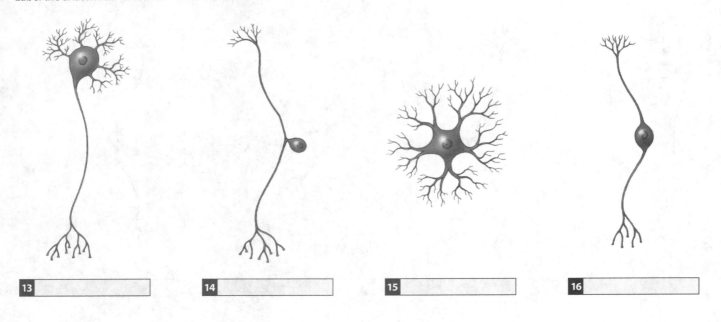

| 13 | | 14 | | 15 | | 16 | |

Vocabulary

In the space provided, write the boldfaced terms introduced in this section that contain the indicated word part.

17	neur- *(nerve)*	17	_____
18	dendr- *(tree)*	18	_____
19	ef- *(away from)*	19	_____
20	af- *(toward)*	20	_____

Vocabulary

Write the term for each of the following descriptions in the space provided.

1. A propagated change in the membrane potential

2. A synapse in which the presynaptic and postsynaptic neuronal membranes are locked together by gap junctions

3. The membrane potential of an unstimulated cell

4. Ion channels that open or close in response to specific stimuli

5. Chemical synapses that release acetylcholine

6. A shift in the membrane potential from -70 mV to -85 mV

7. Movement of positive charges parallel to the inner and outer plasma membrane surfaces

8. A shift in the membrane potential from -70 mV to $+30$ mV

1	_____
2	_____
3	_____
4	_____
5	_____
6	_____
7	_____
8	_____

Short answer

For the following diagram of a cholinergic synapse, write the names of components 9–14 in the boxes at left, and then fill in the table at right with descriptions of the events represented by 15–20.

Components

9	
10	
11	
12	
13	
14	

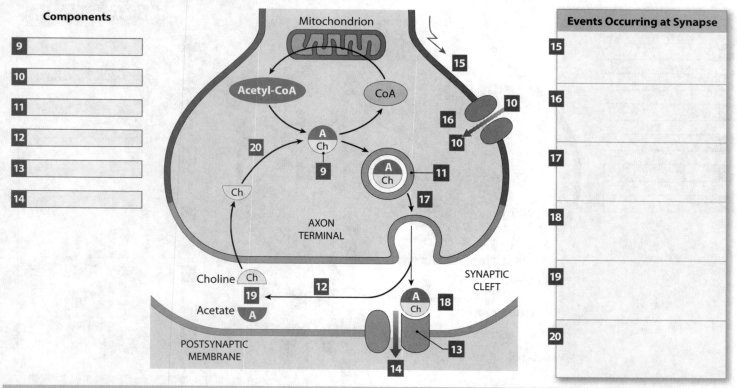

Events Occurring at Synapse

15	
16	
17	
18	
19	
20	

Section integration

Guillain-Barré (GHEE-yan BAH-rā) syndrome is a degeneration of myelin sheaths that ultimately may result in paralysis. Propose a mechanism by which myelin sheath degeneration can cause muscular paralysis.

21. _____

_____

Vocabulary

Write the term for each of the following descriptions in the space provided.

1 A propagated change in the membrane potential

2 A synapse in which the presynaptic and postsynaptic neuronal membranes are locked together by gap junctions

3 The membrane potential of an unstimulated cell

4 Ion channels that open or close in response to specific stimuli

5 Chemical synapses that release acetylcholine

6 A shift in the membrane potential from −70 mV to −85 mV

7 Movement of positive charges parallel to the inner and outer plasma membrane surfaces

8 A shift in the membrane potential from −70 mV to +30 mV

1 _____

2 _____

3 _____

4 _____

5 _____

6 _____

7 _____

8 _____

Short answer

For the following diagram of a cholinergic synapse, write the names of components 9–14 in the boxes at left, and then fill in the table at right with descriptions of the events represented by 15–20.

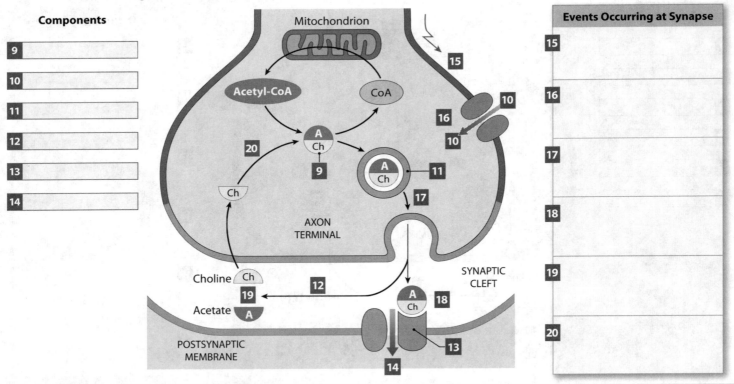

Components

9 _____

10 _____

11 _____

12 _____

13 _____

14 _____

Events Occurring at Synapse
15
16
17
18
19
20

Section integration

Guillain-Barré *(GHEE-yan BAH-rā)* syndrome is a degeneration of myelin sheaths that ultimately may result in paralysis. Propose a mechanism by which myelin sheath degeneration can cause muscular paralysis.

21 _____

_____

Chapter Review Questions

Labeling

Label the structures in the following diagram.

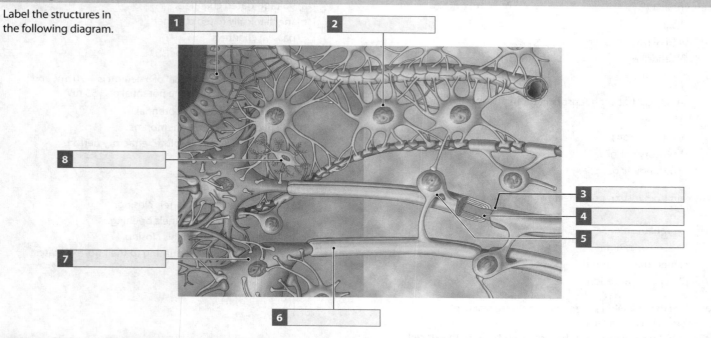

1 [   ]   2 [   ]

8 [   ]

3 [   ]
4 [   ]
5 [   ]

7 [   ]

6 [   ]

True/False

Indicate whether each statement is true or false.

9 Somatic sensory receptors monitor internal organs.

10 Synaptic vesicles contain neurotransmitters.

11 Microglia maintain the blood–brain barrier.

12 Schwann cells form the neurilemma.

13 The resting membrane potential for a neuron is near −70 mV.

9 _____

10 _____

11 _____

12 _____

13 _____

Matching

Match each lettered term with the most closely related description.

a. relative refractory period

b. voltage-gated channel

c. oligodendrocyte

d. chemically gated channel

e. mechanically gated channel

f. Schwann cell

g. absolute refractory period

h. astrocyte

14 Produces myelin in the CNS

15 Opens in response to physical distortion

16 A time when a membrane can respond only to a larger-than-normal stimulus

17 Opens or closes in response to changes in membrane potential

18 Produces myelin in the PNS

19 A time when a membrane cannot respond to further stimulation

20 Maintains the blood–brain barrier

21 Opens in response to neurotransmitters

14 _____

15 _____

16 _____

17 _____

18 _____

19 _____

20 _____

21 _____

Multiple choice

Select the correct answer from the list provided.

22 In the CNS, a neuron typically receives information from other neurons at its

- ☐ a) axon.
- ☐ b) Nissl bodies.
- ☐ c) dendrites.
- ☐ d) nucleus.

23 The neural cells between sensory neurons and motor neurons are

- ☐ a) neuroglia.
- ☐ b) interneurons.
- ☐ c) sensory ganglia.
- ☐ d) autonomic ganglia.

24 Any shift from resting potential toward a more positive value is called

- ☐ a) repolarization.
- ☐ b) depolarization.
- ☐ c) membrane potential.
- ☐ d) hyperpolarization.

25 Which of the following statements is true regarding plasma membrane leak channels?

- ☐ a) Na^+ passively moves through leak channels to exit cell.
- ☐ b) Na^+ actively moves through leak channels to exit cell.
- ☐ c) K^+ passively moves through leak channels to exit cell.
- ☐ d) K^+ actively moves through leak channels to exit cell.

26 Receptors that bind to ACh at the postsynaptic membrane are

- ☐ a) voltage-gated channels.
- ☐ b) mechanically gated channels.
- ☐ c) passive channels.
- ☐ d) chemically gated channels.

27 If the resting membrane potential of a neuron is −70 mV, and threshold is −60 mV, a membrane potential of −55 mV

- ☐ a) will produce an action potential.
- ☐ b) will hyperpolarize the membrane.
- ☐ c) is referred to as the absolute refractory period.
- ☐ d) will cause an IPSP.

28 Repolarization does not include

- ☐ a) voltage-gated Na^+ channels closing.
- ☐ b) voltage-gated Na^+ channels opening.
- ☐ c) voltage-gated K^+ channels closing.
- ☐ d) Na^+ and K^+ channels returning to their normal states.

Short answer

29 What are the major components of the central nervous system (CNS) and the peripheral nervous system (PNS)?

_____

_____

30 What three functional classes of neurons are found in the nervous system? What is the function of each type of neuron?

_____

_____

31 Distinguish between continuous propagation and saltatory propagation.

_____

_____

32 How does a graded potential differ from an action potential?

_____

_____

33 What is the difference between temporal summation and spatial summation?

_____

_____

Labeling

Label each of the structures in the following cross-sectional diagram of the spinal cord.

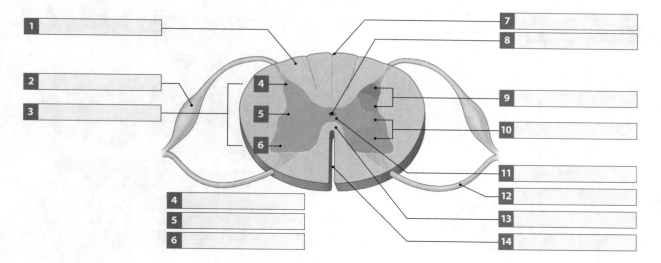

1 _____

2 _____

3 _____

4 ____

5 ____

6 ____

4 _____

5 _____

6 _____

7 _____

8 _____

9 _____

10 _____

11 _____

12 _____

13 _____

14 _____

Label the views (15, 19) and the nerves that innervate the indicated regions of the hands (16–18).

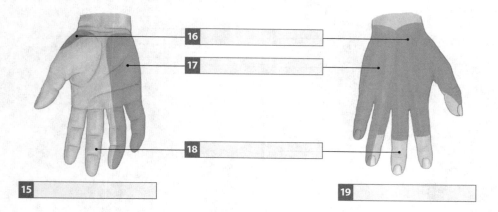
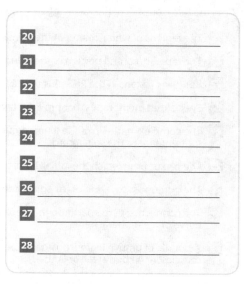

16 _____

17 _____

18 _____

15 _____

19 _____

Vocabulary

Write the term for each of the following descriptions in the space provided.

20 The regions of white matter in the spinal cord

21 The tapered, conical portion of the spinal cord inferior to the lumbar enlargement

22 Bundles of axons in the PNS plus their associated blood vessels and connective tissues

23 Specialized membranes that provide stability and support for the spinal cord and brain

24 The complex made up of the filum terminale and the long dorsal and ventral spinal nerve roots inferior to the spinal cord

25 The plexus from which the radial, median, and ulnar nerves originate

26 The outermost covering of the spinal cord

27 The connective tissue partition that separates adjacent bundles of nerve fibers in a spinal nerve or a peripheral nerve

28 A bundle of unmyelinated, postganglionic fibers that innervates glands and smooth muscles in the body wall or limbs

20 _____

21 _____

22 _____

23 _____

24 _____

25 _____

26 _____

27 _____

28 _____

Labeling

Label each of the structures in the following cross-sectional diagram of the spinal cord.

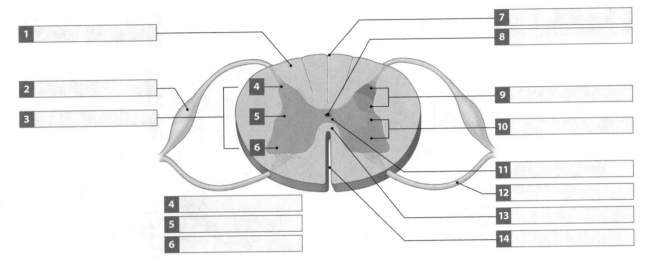

1		7	
		8	
2			
3		9	
		10	
4		11	
5		12	
6		13	
		14	

Label the views (15, 19) and the nerves that innervate the indicated regions of the hands (16–18).

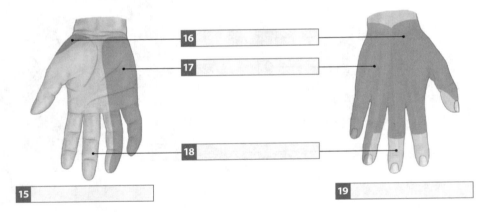

16	
17	
18	
15	
19	

Vocabulary

Write the term for each of the following descriptions in the space provided.

20 The regions of white matter in the spinal cord

21 The tapered, conical portion of the spinal cord inferior to the lumbar enlargement

22 Bundles of axons in the PNS plus their associated blood vessels and connective tissues

23 Specialized membranes that provide stability and support for the spinal cord and brain

24 The complex made up of the filum terminale and the long dorsal and ventral spinal nerve roots inferior to the spinal cord

25 The plexus from which the radial, median, and ulnar nerves originate

26 The outermost covering of the spinal cord

27 The connective tissue partition that separates adjacent bundles of nerve fibers in a spinal nerve or a peripheral nerve

28 A bundle of unmyelinated, postganglionic fibers that innervates glands and smooth muscles in the body wall or limbs

20 _____

21 _____

22 _____

23 _____

24 _____

25 _____

26 _____

27 _____

28 _____

Labeling

Label the neural circuit patterns in the following diagrams.

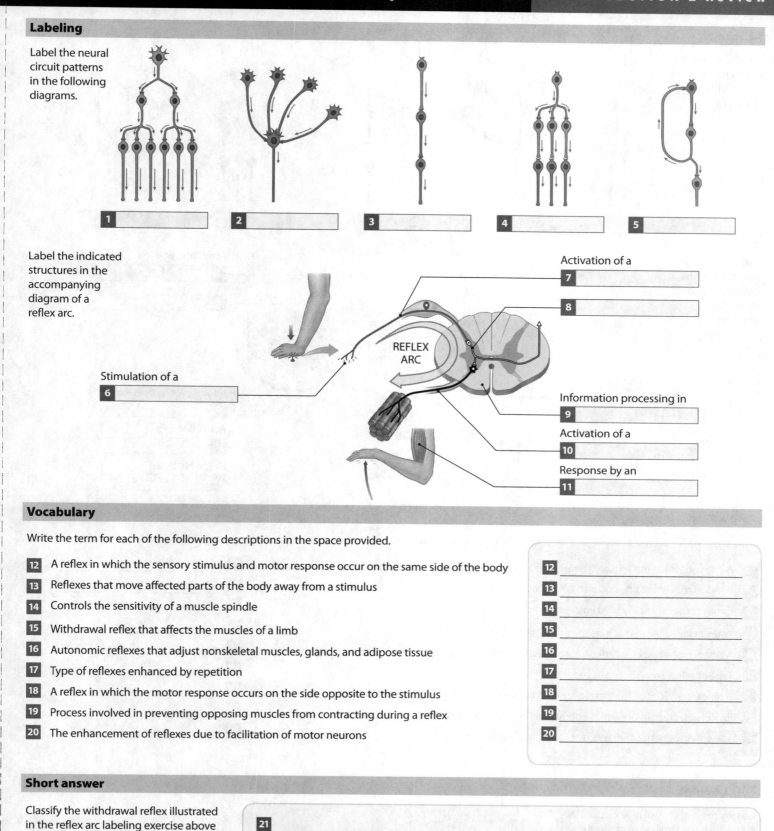

| 1 | | 2 | | 3 | | 4 | | 5 | |

Label the indicated structures in the accompanying diagram of a reflex arc.

REFLEX ARC

Stimulation of a
6

Activation of a
7

8

Information processing in
9

Activation of a
10

Response by an
11

Vocabulary

Write the term for each of the following descriptions in the space provided.

12 A reflex in which the sensory stimulus and motor response occur on the same side of the body

13 Reflexes that move affected parts of the body away from a stimulus

14 Controls the sensitivity of a muscle spindle

15 Withdrawal reflex that affects the muscles of a limb

16 Autonomic reflexes that adjust nonskeletal muscles, glands, and adipose tissue

17 Type of reflexes enhanced by repetition

18 A reflex in which the motor response occurs on the side opposite to the stimulus

19 Process involved in preventing opposing muscles from contracting during a reflex

20 The enhancement of reflexes due to facilitation of motor neurons

12 _____

13 _____

14 _____

15 _____

16 _____

17 _____

18 _____

19 _____

20 _____

Short answer

Classify the withdrawal reflex illustrated in the reflex arc labeling exercise above according to development, response, complexity of circuit, and processing site.

21 _____
_____
_____

93

Labeling

Label the neural circuit patterns in the following diagrams.

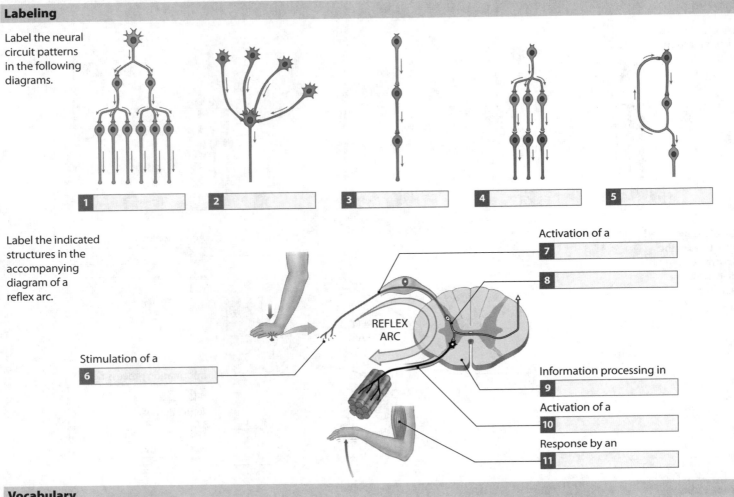

1 _____

2 _____

3 _____

4 _____

5 _____

Label the indicated structures in the accompanying diagram of a reflex arc.

Activation of a
7 _____

8 _____

REFLEX ARC

Stimulation of a
6 _____

Information processing in
9 _____

Activation of a
10 _____

Response by an
11 _____

Vocabulary

Write the term for each of the following descriptions in the space provided.

12 A reflex in which the sensory stimulus and motor response occur on the same side of the body

13 Reflexes that move affected parts of the body away from a stimulus

14 Controls the sensitivity of a muscle spindle

15 Withdrawal reflex that affects the muscles of a limb

16 Autonomic reflexes that adjust nonskeletal muscles, glands, and adipose tissue

17 Type of reflexes enhanced by repetition

18 A reflex in which the motor response occurs on the side opposite to the stimulus

19 Process involved in preventing opposing muscles from contracting during a reflex

20 The enhancement of reflexes due to facilitation of motor neurons

12 _____
13 _____
14 _____
15 _____
16 _____
17 _____
18 _____
19 _____
20 _____

Short answer

Classify the withdrawal reflex illustrated in the reflex arc labeling exercise above according to development, response, complexity of circuit, and processing site.

21 _____
_____
_____

Chapter Review Questions

Labeling

Label the structures in the following diagram.

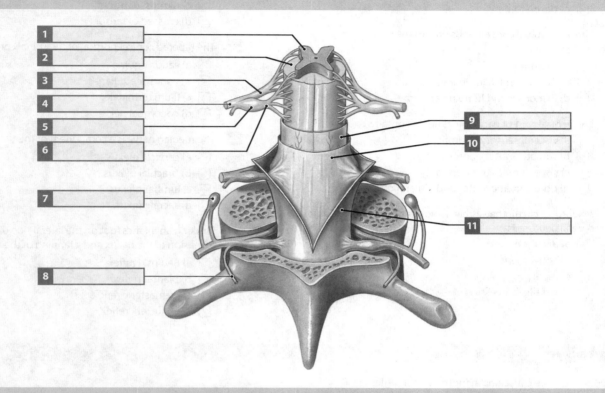

1	
2	
3	
4	
5	
6	
7	
8	
9	
10	
11	

True/False

Indicate whether each statement is true or false.

12 Sensory input travels toward the spinal cord and motor commands travel away from the spinal cord.

13 Endoneurium is the outermost covering of a spinal nerve.

14 The dorsal root of each spinal nerve carries motor information away from the spinal cord.

15 There are eight cervical spinal nerves.

16 Motor nuclei are located in the posterior gray horn of the spinal cord.

12	_____
13	_____
14	_____
15	_____
16	_____

Multiple choice

Select the correct answer from the list provided.

17 The following steps are involved in a simple neural reflex: (1) activation of a sensory neuron; (2) activation of a motor neuron; (3) response of a peripheral effector; (4) a stimulus activates a receptor; (5) information processing. The proper sequence of these steps is

- ☐ a) 1, 3, 4, 5, 2.
- ☐ b) 4, 5, 3, 1, 2.
- ☐ c) 4, 1, 5, 2, 3.
- ☐ d) 4, 3, 1, 5, 2.

18 The layers of the spinal meninges from superficial to deep are

- ☐ a) pia mater, arachnoid, dura mater.
- ☐ b) arachnoid, pia mater, dura mater.
- ☐ c) dura mater, arachnoid, pia mater.
- ☐ d) dura mater, pia mater, arachnoid.

19 Fascicles containing bundles of axons are surrounded by
- ☐ a) epineurium.
- ☐ b) perineurium.
- ☐ c) endoneurium.
- ☐ d) dermatome.

20 The adult spinal cord extends only to the
- ☐ a) coccyx.
- ☐ b) sacrum.
- ☐ c) third or fourth lumbar vertebra.
- ☐ d) first or second lumbar vertebra.

21 The ventral root of each spinal nerve contains axons of
- ☐ a) visceral sensory neurons.
- ☐ b) somatic motor neurons only.
- ☐ c) visceral motor neurons only.
- ☐ d) both somatic motor and visceral motor neurons.

22 A neuronal circuit that spreads information from one neuron to several neurons is
- ☐ a) divergence.
- ☐ b) convergence.
- ☐ c) serial processing.
- ☐ d) parallel processing.

23 Reflex arcs in which the sensory stimulus and the motor response occur on the same side of the body are
- ☐ a) contralateral.
- ☐ b) ipsilateral.
- ☐ c) monosynaptic.
- ☐ d) crossed extensor.

24 The tapered conical portion of the spinal cord is the
- ☐ a) cauda equina.
- ☐ b) conus medullaris.
- ☐ c) filum terminale.
- ☐ d) coccygeal nerve.

25 The median nerve is a component of the
- ☐ a) cervical plexus.
- ☐ b) brachial plexus.
- ☐ c) lumbar plexus.
- ☐ d) sacral plexus.

26 Stroking an infant's foot on the lateral side of the sole produces extension of the hallux and a fanning of the toes known as the
- ☐ a) Babinski reflex.
- ☐ b) plantar reflex.
- ☐ c) cremasteric reflex.
- ☐ d) ankle jerk reflex.

Short answer

27 Describe the cause and symptoms of shingles.

_____
_____
_____

28 A student forcefully bumps the posterior medial aspect of her elbow on her desktop and feels pain in her hand. Which nerve is involved, and where in her hand is she experiencing pain?

_____
_____
_____

29 Why do cervical nerves outnumber cervical vertebrae?

_____
_____
_____

30 Where is cerebrospinal fluid located, and what are its functions?

_____
_____
_____
_____

Labeling

Label the structures in the accompanying figure of a lateral view of the human brain.

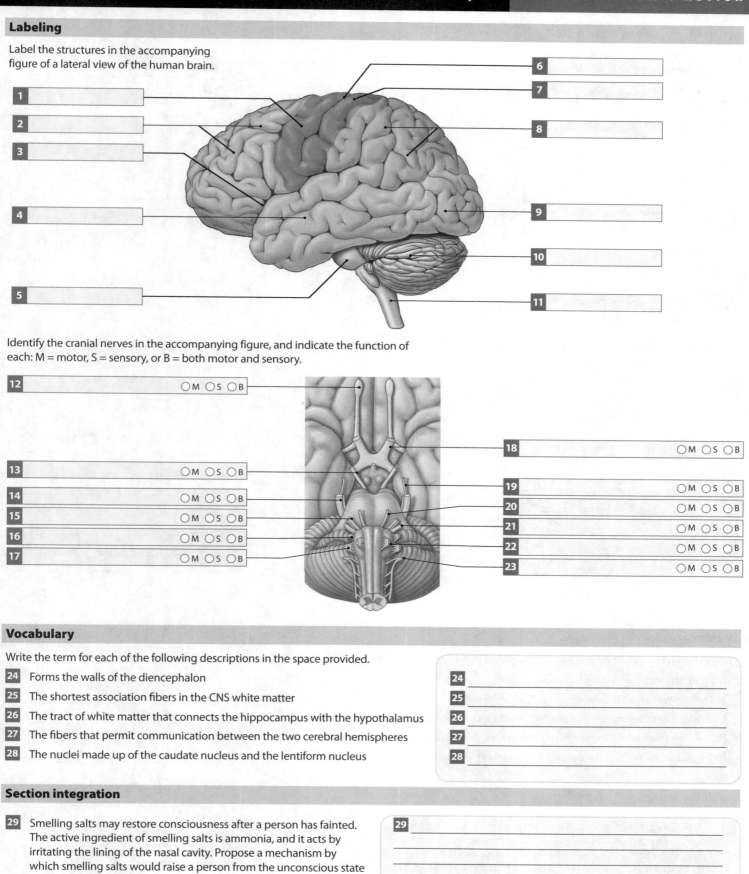

| 1 |
| 2 |
| 3 |
| 4 |
| 5 |

| 6 |
| 7 |
| 8 |
| 9 |
| 10 |
| 11 |

Identify the cranial nerves in the accompanying figure, and indicate the function of each: M = motor, S = sensory, or B = both motor and sensory.

12	○ M ○ S ○ B
13	○ M ○ S ○ B
14	○ M ○ S ○ B
15	○ M ○ S ○ B
16	○ M ○ S ○ B
17	○ M ○ S ○ B

18	○ M ○ S ○ B
19	○ M ○ S ○ B
20	○ M ○ S ○ B
21	○ M ○ S ○ B
22	○ M ○ S ○ B
23	○ M ○ S ○ B

Vocabulary

Write the term for each of the following descriptions in the space provided.

24 Forms the walls of the diencephalon

25 The shortest association fibers in the CNS white matter

26 The tract of white matter that connects the hippocampus with the hypothalamus

27 The fibers that permit communication between the two cerebral hemispheres

28 The nuclei made up of the caudate nucleus and the lentiform nucleus

24 _____

25 _____

26 _____

27 _____

28 _____

Section integration

29 Smelling salts may restore consciousness after a person has fainted. The active ingredient of smelling salts is ammonia, and it acts by irritating the lining of the nasal cavity. Propose a mechanism by which smelling salts would raise a person from the unconscious state to the conscious state.

29 _____

Labeling

Label the structures in the accompanying figure of a lateral view of the human brain.

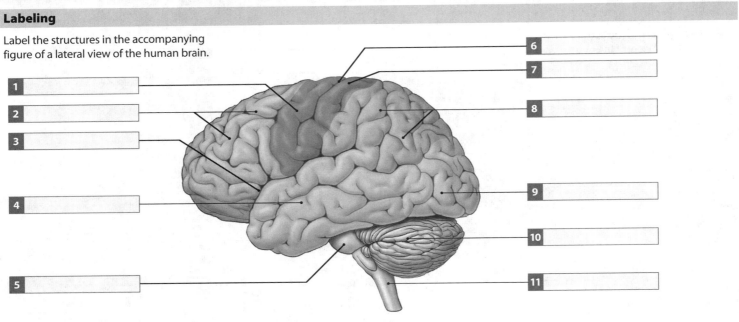

1	6
2	7
3	8
4	9
5	10
	11

Identify the cranial nerves in the accompanying figure, and indicate the function of each: M = motor, S = sensory, or B = both motor and sensory.

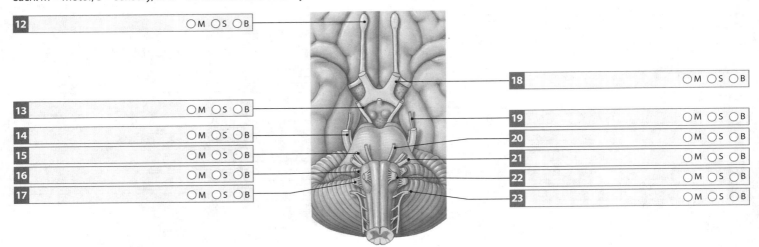

12   ○M ○S ○B

13   ○M ○S ○B

14   ○M ○S ○B

15   ○M ○S ○B

16   ○M ○S ○B

17   ○M ○S ○B

18   ○M ○S ○B

19   ○M ○S ○B

20   ○M ○S ○B

21   ○M ○S ○B

22   ○M ○S ○B

23   ○M ○S ○B

Vocabulary

Write the term for each of the following descriptions in the space provided.

24   Forms the walls of the diencephalon

25   The shortest association fibers in the CNS white matter

26   The tract of white matter that connects the hippocampus with the hypothalamus

27   The fibers that permit communication between the two cerebral hemispheres

28   The nuclei made up of the caudate nucleus and the lentiform nucleus

24 _____

25 _____

26 _____

27 _____

28 _____

Section integration

29   Smelling salts may restore consciousness after a person has fainted. The active ingredient of smelling salts is ammonia, and it acts by irritating the lining of the nasal cavity. Propose a mechanism by which smelling salts would raise a person from the unconscious state to the conscious state.

29 _____

_____

_____

_____

Labeling

Label each type of tactile receptor found in the skin.

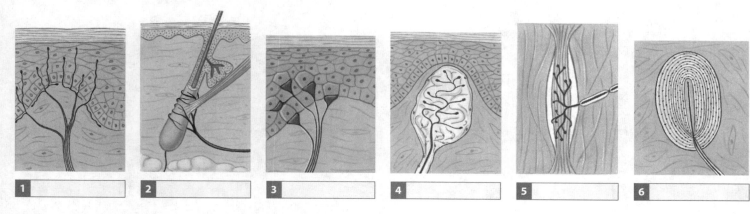

1	2	3	4	5	6

Fill-in

The general organization of the spinal cord is such that motor tracts are [7 _____] (anterior or posterior), and sensory tracts are [8 _____] (anterior or posterior).

Short answer

Identify the descending and ascending tracts and pathways in the accompanying sectional diagram of the spinal cord, and then describe the general functions of the tracts of each pathway.

| 9 |
| 10 |
| 11 |
| 12 |
| 13 |
| 14 |

| 15 |
| 16 |
| 17 |
| 18 |
| 19 |

Section integration

A person whose primary motor cortex has been injured retains the ability to walk, maintain balance, and perform other voluntary and involuntary movements. Even though the movements lack precision and are awkward and poorly controlled, why is the ability to walk and maintain balance possible?

| 20 _____ |

Labeling

Label each type of tactile receptor found in the skin.

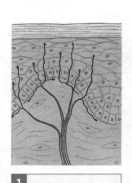 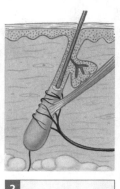 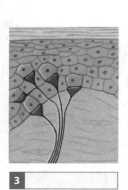 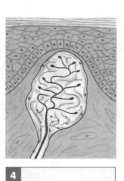 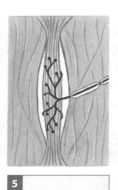 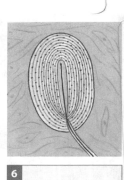

1 _____
2 _____
3 _____
4 _____
5 _____
6 _____

Fill-in

The general organization of the spinal cord is such that motor tracts are [7] _____ (anterior or posterior),

and sensory tracts are [8] _____ (anterior or posterior).

Short answer

Identify the descending and ascending tracts and pathways in the accompanying sectional
diagram of the spinal cord, and then describe the general functions of the tracts of each pathway.

9 _____

10 _____

11 _____

12 _____

13 _____

14 _____

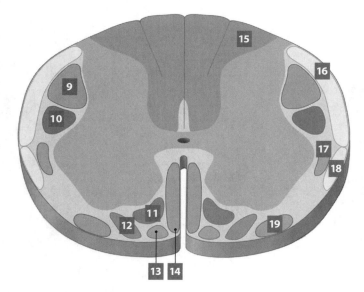

15 _____

16 _____

17 _____

18 _____

19 _____

Section integration

A person whose primary motor cortex has been injured retains the ability to walk, maintain balance, and perform other voluntary and involuntary
movements. Even though the movements lack precision and are awkward and poorly controlled, why is the ability to walk and maintain balance
possible?

20 _____

_____

Chapter Review Questions

Labeling

Label the structures of the brain indicated in the following diagram.

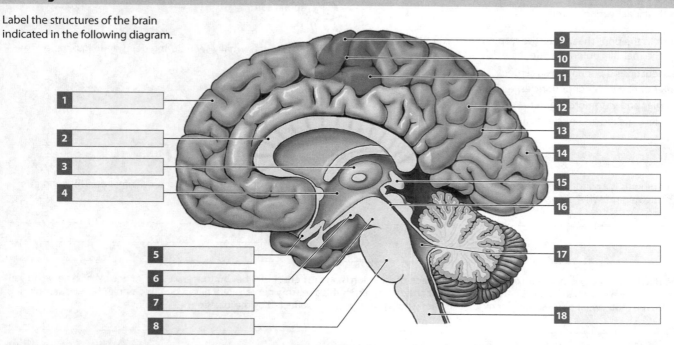

1. _____
2. _____
3. _____
4. _____
5. _____
6. _____
7. _____
8. _____
9. _____
10. _____
11. _____
12. _____
13. _____
14. _____
15. _____
16. _____
17. _____
18. _____

True/False

Indicate whether each statement is true or false.

19. The special sensory cranial nerves are I, II, VIII, and X.
20. Proprioceptors are the general sensory receptors that monitor the positions of joints and muscles.
21. Parkinson's disease is characterized by demyelination that affects axons of the optic nerve, brain, and spinal cord.
22. Ruffini corpuscles are often referred to as free nerve endings.
23. The posterior column pathway carries sensations of touch, pressure, vibration, and proprioception.

19. _____
20. _____
21. _____
22. _____
23. _____

Multiple choice

Select the correct answer from the list provided.

24. The adult cerebrum develops from the
    - a) diencephalon.
    - b) telencephalon.
    - c) mesencephalon.
    - d) metencephalon.

25. The cerebral aqueduct connects the
    - a) lateral ventricles to the third ventricle.
    - b) third ventricle to the fourth ventricle.
    - c) fourth ventricle to the central canal.
    - d) lateral ventricles to the interventricular foramen.

26. The fold of dura mater that projects between the cerebral hemispheres is the
    - a) falx cerebri.
    - b) falx cerebelli.
    - c) tentorium cerebelli.
    - d) superior sagittal sinus.

27. The leading site where CSF is absorbed into venous circulation is the
    - a) lateral apertures.
    - b) median aperture.
    - c) choroid plexuses.
    - d) arachnoid granulations.

28 The superior and inferior colliculi collectively form the

☐ a) thalamus.

☐ b) corpora quadrigemina.

☐ c) limbic system.

☐ d) reticular activating system.

29 The centers in the pons that adjust the respiratory rhythmicity centers in the medulla oblongata are the

☐ a) apneustic and pneumotaxic centers.

☐ b) inferior and superior peduncles.

☐ c) cardiac and vasomotor centers

☐ d) nucleus gracilis and nucleus cuneatus.

30 The final relay point for ascending sensory information that will be projected to the primary sensory cortex is the

☐ a) hypothalamus.

☐ b) thalamus.

☐ c) spinal cord.

☐ d) pons.

31 The brain waves normally seen during deep sleep in people of all ages are called

☐ a) alpha waves.

☐ b) beta waves.

☐ c) theta waves.

☐ d) delta waves.

Short answer

32 Cerebral meningitis is a condition in which the meninges of the brain become inflamed as the result of viral or bacterial infection. This condition can be life threatening. Why?

_____

_____

_____

33 Julia is about to have a cavity in her tooth filled. The tooth in need of attention is on the right side of her bottom jaw in the far back. Which nerve do you think the dentist will block when he gives her an injection to control the pain? Is this a sensory nerve, motor nerve, or mixed nerve? Besides stopping the pain from the tooth, what other sensory or motor activities would you expect to be affected by the injection?

_____

_____

_____

Labeling

Fill in the missing labels in this diagram of the sympathetic division of the ANS.

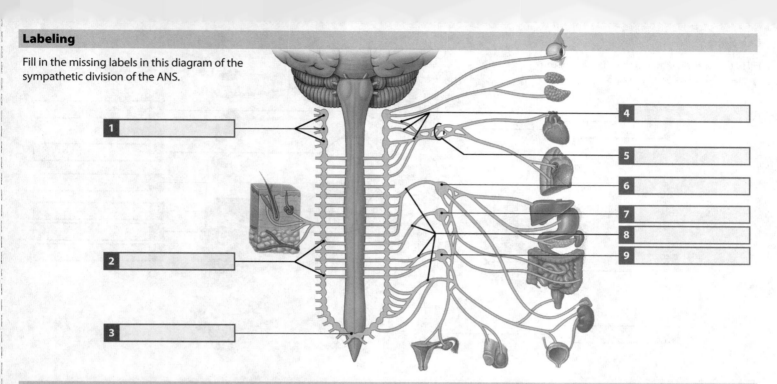

1 _____
2 _____
3 _____
4 _____
5 _____
6 _____
7 _____
8 _____
9 _____

Concept map

Use each of the following terms once to fill in the blank boxes to correctly complete the map.

- sympathetic division
- craniosacral division
- cranial nerves III, VII, IX, X
- thoracolumbar division
- parasympathetic division
- sacral nerves
- thoracic nerves
- enteric nervous system
- lumbar nerves

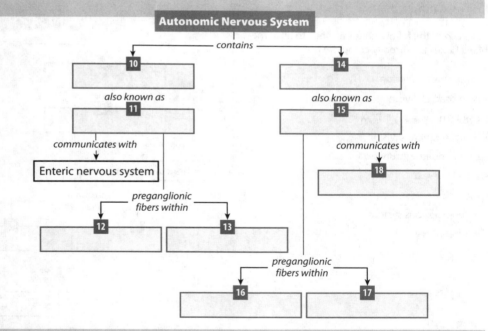

Autonomic Nervous System

contains

10 _____

also known as

11 _____

communicates with

Enteric nervous system

preganglionic fibers within

12 _____   13 _____

14 _____

also known as

15 _____

communicates with

18 _____

preganglionic fibers within

16 _____   17 _____

Matching

Match each lettered term with the most closely related description.

a. nicotinic, muscarinic
b. secrete norepinephrine
c. receptors
d. alpha, beta
e. cholinergic
f. splanchnic nerves
g. acetylcholine
h. parasympathetic activation

19 Collateral ganglia
20 Parasympathetic neurotransmitter
21 Sexual arousal
22 Adrenal medullae
23 Cholinergic receptors
24 Determines neurotransmitter effects
25 All parasympathetic neurons
26 Adrenergic receptors

19 _____
20 _____
21 _____
22 _____
23 _____
24 _____
25 _____
26 _____

Labeling

Fill in the missing labels in this diagram of the sympathetic division of the ANS.

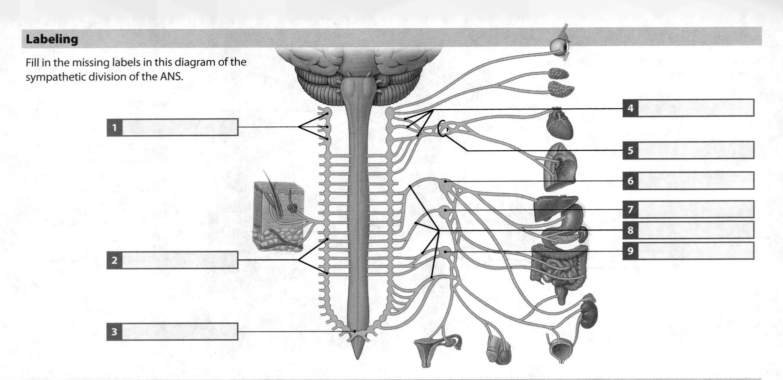

1
2
3
4
5
6
7
8
9

Concept map

Use each of the following terms once to fill in the blank boxes to correctly complete the map.

- sympathetic division
- craniosacral division
- cranial nerves III, VII, IX, X
- thoracolumbar division
- parasympathetic division
- sacral nerves
- thoracic nerves
- enteric nervous system
- lumbar nerves

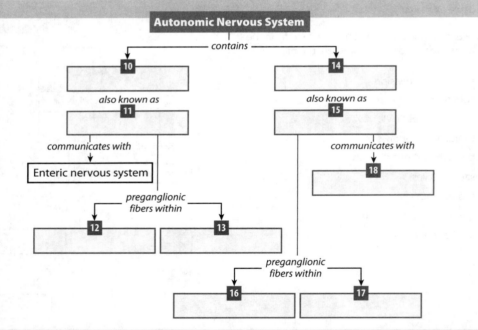

Autonomic Nervous System

— *contains* —

10

also known as
11

communicates with

Enteric nervous system

preganglionic fibers within

12   13

14

also known as
15

communicates with
18

preganglionic fibers within

16   17

Matching

Match each lettered term with the most closely related description.

a. nicotinic, muscarinic
b. secrete norepinephrine
c. receptors
d. alpha, beta
e. cholinergic
f. splanchnic nerves
g. acetylcholine
h. parasympathetic activation

19 Collateral ganglia
20 Parasympathetic neurotransmitter
21 Sexual arousal
22 Adrenal medullae
23 Cholinergic receptors
24 Determines neurotransmitter effects
25 All parasympathetic neurons
26 Adrenergic receptors

19 _____
20 _____
21 _____
22 _____
23 _____
24 _____
25 _____
26 _____

Concept map

Use each of the following terms once to fill in the blank boxes to correctly complete the map.

- respiratory
- pons
- spinal cord T$_1$–L$_2$
- vasomotor
- coughing
- hypothalamus
- sympathetic visceral reflexes
- parasympathetic visceral reflexes
- complex visceral reflexes
- limbic system and thalamus

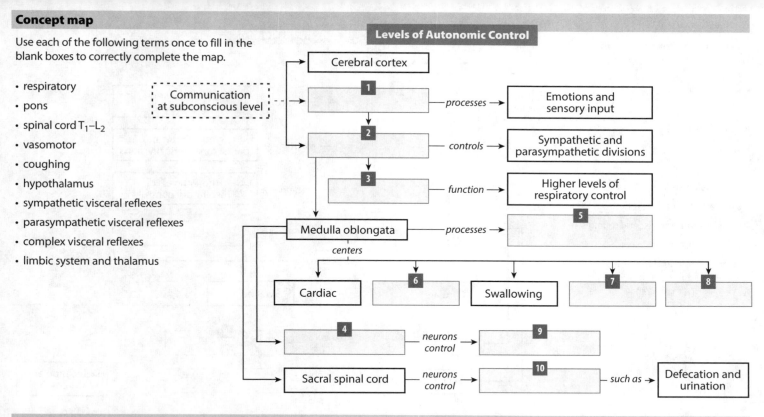

Levels of Autonomic Control

Cerebral cortex

1 → *processes* → Emotions and sensory input

2 → *controls* → Sympathetic and parasympathetic divisions

3 → *function* → Higher levels of respiratory control

Communication at subconscious level

Medulla oblongata → *processes* → 5

centers

Cardiac   6   Swallowing   7   8

4 → *neurons control* → 9

Sacral spinal cord → *neurons control* → 10 → *such as* → Defecation and urination

Fill-in

Fill in S (sympathetic) or P (parasympathetic) to indicate the ANS division responsible for each of the following effects.

11	Decreased metabolic rate	11 ○ S ○ P
12	Increased salivary and digestive secretions	12 ○ S ○ P
13	Increased metabolic rate	13 ○ S ○ P
14	Stimulation of urination and defecation	14 ○ S ○ P
15	Activation of sweat glands	15 ○ S ○ P
16	Heightened mental alertness	16 ○ S ○ P
17	Decreased heart rate and blood pressure	17 ○ S ○ P
18	Activation of energy reserves	18 ○ S ○ P
19	Increased heart rate and blood pressure	19 ○ S ○ P
20	Reduced digestive and urinary functions	20 ○ S ○ P
21	Increased motility and blood flow in the digestive tract	21 ○ S ○ P
22	Increased respiratory rate and dilation of respiratory passages	22 ○ S ○ P
23	Constriction of the pupils and focus of the eyes on nearby objects	23 ○ S ○ P

Short answer

Recent surveys show that about one-third of the American adult population is involved in some type of exercise program. What contributions does sympathetic activation make to help the body adjust to changes that occur during exercise and still maintain homeostasis?

24 _____

_____

Concept map

Use each of the following terms once to fill in the blank boxes to correctly complete the map.

- respiratory
- pons
- spinal cord T_1–L_2
- vasomotor
- coughing
- hypothalamus
- sympathetic visceral reflexes
- parasympathetic visceral reflexes
- complex visceral reflexes
- limbic system and thalamus

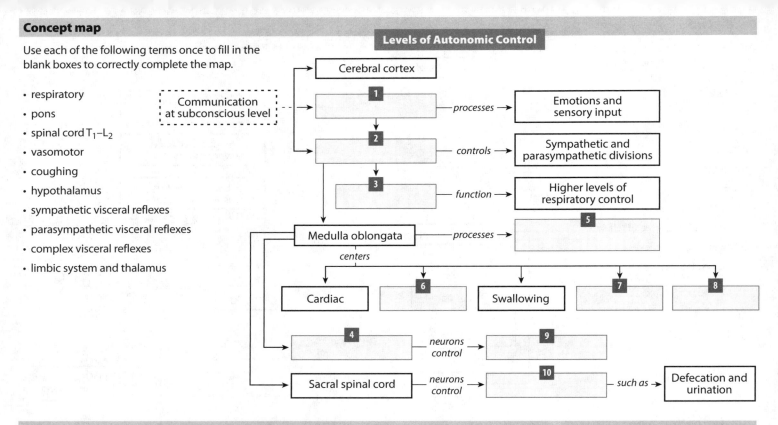

Levels of Autonomic Control

Cerebral cortex

1 ── *processes* → Emotions and sensory input

Communication at subconscious level

2 ── *controls* → Sympathetic and parasympathetic divisions

3 ── *function* → Higher levels of respiratory control

Medulla oblongata ── *processes* → 5

centers

Cardiac | 6 | Swallowing | 7 | 8

4 ── *neurons control* → 9

Sacral spinal cord ── *neurons control* → 10 ── *such as* → Defecation and urination

Fill-in

Fill in S (sympathetic) or P (parasympathetic) to indicate the ANS division responsible for each of the following effects.

11 Decreased metabolic rate   11 ○ S ○ P

12 Increased salivary and digestive secretions   12 ○ S ○ P

13 Increased metabolic rate   13 ○ S ○ P

14 Stimulation of urination and defecation   14 ○ S ○ P

15 Activation of sweat glands   15 ○ S ○ P

16 Heightened mental alertness   16 ○ S ○ P

17 Decreased heart rate and blood pressure   17 ○ S ○ P

18 Activation of energy reserves   18 ○ S ○ P

19 Increased heart rate and blood pressure   19 ○ S ○ P

20 Reduced digestive and urinary functions   20 ○ S ○ P

21 Increased motility and blood flow in the digestive tract   21 ○ S ○ P

22 Increased respiratory rate and dilation of respiratory passages   22 ○ S ○ P

23 Constriction of the pupils and focus of the eyes on nearby objects   23 ○ S ○ P

Short answer

Recent surveys show that about one-third of the American adult population is involved in some type of exercise program. What contributions does sympathetic activation make to help the body adjust to changes that occur during exercise and still maintain homeostasis?

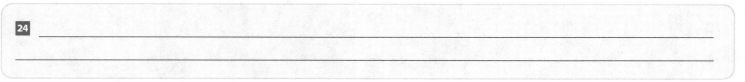

24 _____

_____

Chapter Review Questions

Labeling

Label the anatomical characteristics of the ANS shown in the diagram below.

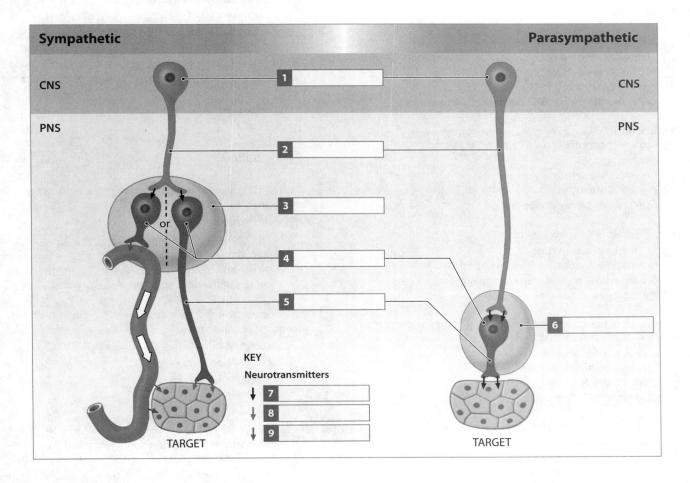

True/False

Indicate whether each statement is true or false.

10 Ganglionic neurons have their cell bodies in the CNS.

11 The enteric nervous system is influenced by both the sympathetic and parasympathetic divisions.

12 The celiac ganglion is associated with sympathetic regulation of the cardiovascular and respiratory systems.

13 All effector organs receive dual innervation.

14 Chemoreceptors of the carotid and aortic bodies are sensitive to changes in blood pressure.

15 Nicotinic receptors can be found at the neuromuscular junctions of skeletal muscle fibers.

10 _____

11 _____

12 _____

13 _____

14 _____

15 _____

Multiple choice

Select the correct answer from the list provided.

16 Which of the following is *not* a visceral effector?
- a) smooth muscle
- b) glands
- c) skeletal muscle
- d) adipocytes

17 Sympathetic division axons emerge from
- a) the brain stem and the sacral segments of the spinal cord.
- b) cranial nerves III, VIII, IX, and X.
- c) only sacral nerves.
- d) the thoracic nerves and lumbar nerves L_1 and L_2.

18 Which of the following ganglionic neurons synapse with preganglionic fibers of the parasympathetic division?
- a) ciliary ganglia
- b) sympathetic chain
- c) adrenal medulla
- d) inferior mesenteric ganglia

19 The autonomic nervous system directs
- a) voluntary motor activity.
- b) conscious control of skeletal muscles.
- c) unconscious processes that maintain homeostasis.
- d) sensory input from the skin.

20 The division of the autonomic nervous system that prepares the body for activity and stress is the
- a) sympathetic division.
- b) parasympathetic division.
- c) enteric division.
- d) somatomotor division.

21 The two types of cholinergic receptors are
- a) alpha-1 and alpha-2 receptors.
- b) beta-1 and beta-2 receptors.
- c) nicotinic and muscarinic receptors.
- d) alpha-1 and beta-1 receptors.

22 Which receptors would you block to cause a decreased heart rate?
- a) alpha-1 receptors
- b) beta-1 receptors
- c) nicotinic receptors
- d) muscarinic receptors

23 Where are the chemoreceptors found that are sensitive to changes in pH and P_{CO_2} in arterial blood?
- a) carotid and aortic bodies
- b) carotid and aortic sinuses
- c) baroreceptors of the lungs
- d) respiratory centers of the medulla oblongata

24 A drug that stimulates which receptor would relax the smooth muscle passages and increase airway diameter of the respiratory tract?
- a) beta-1
- b) beta-2
- c) beta-3
- d) muscarinic

25 Which of the following responses is *not* characteristic of sympathetic activation?
- a) increased alertness
- b) elevation of muscle tone
- c) erection
- d) increased activity in the cardiovascular and respiratory centers of the pons and medulla oblongata

26 Which neurotransmitter is released by all preganglionic fibers of the autonomic nervous system?
- a) acetylcholine
- b) epinephrine
- c) norepinephrine
- d) serotonin

27 Dual innervation refers to situations in which vital organs
- a) receive information from both sympathetic and parasympathetic fibers.
- b) receive information from both the somatic and autonomic nervous systems.
- c) are receptive to multiple neurotransmitters.
- d) are under both conscious and unconscious control.

Short answer

28 Identify the components of a visceral reflex arc, and distinguish between short reflexes and long reflexes.

29 Identify at least three differences between the somatic and autonomic nervous systems.

30 Which cranial and sacral nerves are associated with the parasympathetic division?

Labeling

Label taste sensations associated with areas on the tongue (1–5) and the four types of lingual papillae (6–9).

1 _____

2 _____

3 _____

4 _____

5 _____

6 _____

7 _____

8 _____

9 _____

Matching

Match each lettered term with the most closely related description.

a. gustation
b. depolarization
c. Bowman's glands
d. lingual papillae
e. G proteins
f. stem cells
g. bitter
h. olfactory dendrites
i. olfaction
j. taste bud
k. cerebral cortex
l. olfactory bulb
m. odorant

10 Sweet, bitter, and umami sensations
11 Sense of smell
12 Basal cells
13 Chemical stimulus
14 Sense of taste
15 Olfactory glands
16 Receives all special senses stimuli
17 Cluster of gustatory receptors
18 Site of first synapse by olfactory receptors
19 Contain olfactory receptor proteins
20 Most sensitive taste sensation
21 Produces generator potential
22 Epithelial projections of tongue

10 _____
11 _____
12 _____
13 _____
14 _____
15 _____
16 _____
17 _____
18 _____
19 _____
20 _____
21 _____
22 _____

Section integration

Contrast the sensory receptors for olfaction with the sensory receptors for taste, vision, equilibrium, and hearing.

23 _____

_____

_____

Labeling

Label taste sensations associated with areas on the tongue (1–5) and the four types of lingual papillae (6–9).

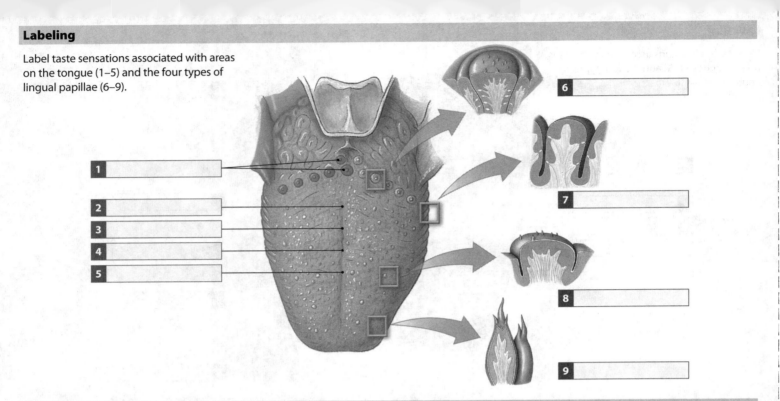

1	
2	
3	
4	
5	

6	
7	
8	
9	

Matching

Match each lettered term with the most closely related description.

a. gustation
b. depolarization
c. Bowman's glands
d. lingual papillae
e. G proteins
f. stem cells
g. bitter
h. olfactory dendrites
i. olfaction
j. taste bud
k. cerebral cortex
l. olfactory bulb
m. odorant

10 Sweet, bitter, and umami sensations
11 Sense of smell
12 Basal cells
13 Chemical stimulus
14 Sense of taste
15 Olfactory glands
16 Receives all special senses stimuli
17 Cluster of gustatory receptors
18 Site of first synapse by olfactory receptors
19 Contain olfactory receptor proteins
20 Most sensitive taste sensation
21 Produces generator potential
22 Epithelial projections of tongue

10	
11	
12	
13	
14	
15	
16	
17	
18	
19	
20	
21	
22	

Section integration

Contrast the sensory receptors for olfaction with the sensory receptors for taste, vision, equilibrium, and hearing.

23	

Labeling

Label the structures in the following diagram of the right ear.

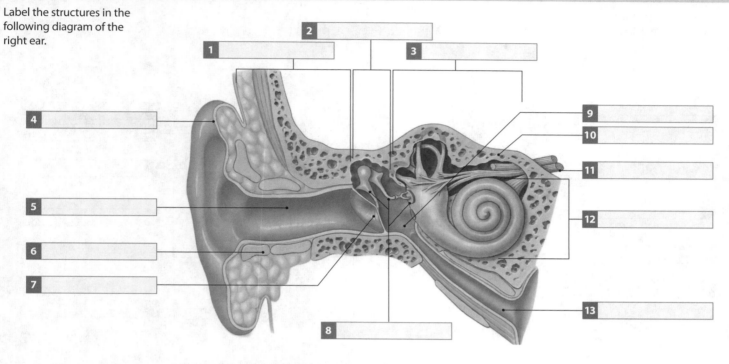

| 1 | | 2 | | 3 | |

4	
5	
6	
7	
8	

9	
10	
11	
12	
13	

Label the structures in the following micrograph of the internal ear.

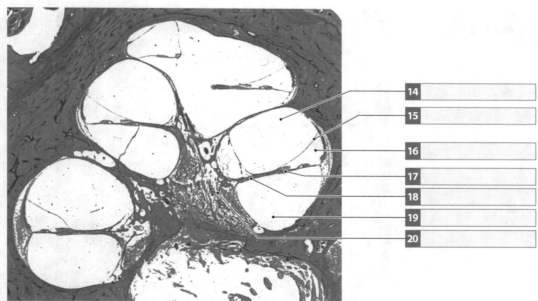

14	
15	
16	
17	
18	
19	
20	

Section integration

For a few seconds after you ride an express elevator from the 25th floor to the ground floor, you still feel as if you are descending, even though you have come to a stop. Why?

21	_____
	_____
	_____

Labeling

Label the structures in the following diagram of the right ear.

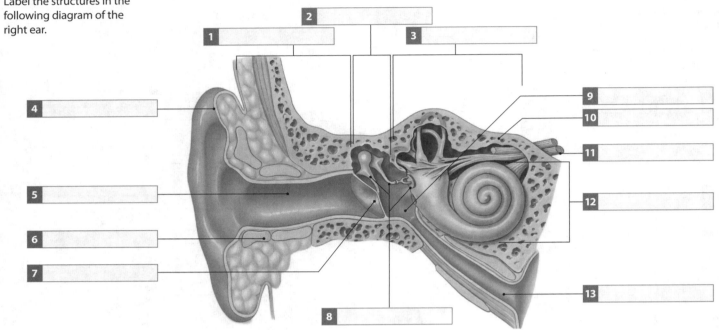

1	
2	
3	
4	
5	
6	
7	
8	
9	
10	
11	
12	
13	

Label the structures in the following micrograph of the internal ear.

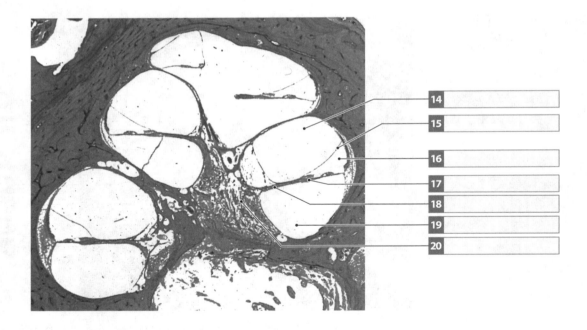

14	
15	
16	
17	
18	
19	
20	

Section integration

For a few seconds after you ride an express elevator from the 25th floor to the ground floor, you still feel as if you are descending, even though you have come to a stop. Why?

21 _____

_____

_____

Labeling

Label the structures in this diagram of a sagittal section of the left eye.

1	
2	
3	
4	
5	
6	
7	

8	
9	
10	
11	
12	
13	
14	
15	
16	

Matching

Match each lettered term with the most closely related description.

a. ganglion cells
b. cones
c. vascular layer
d. rods
e. optic disc
f. posterior chamber
g. crystallins
h. sclera
i. retina
j. occipital lobe
k. palpebrae
l. rhodopsin
m. fovea
n. posterior cavity
o. pupil

17 Visual pigment
18 Eyelids
19 Transparent proteins in the cells of a lens
20 White of the eye
21 Opening surrounded by the iris
22 Inner layer
23 Site of vitreous body
24 Photoreceptors that enable vision in dim light
25 Extends between the iris and the ciliary body and lens
26 Sharpest vision
27 Visual cortex
28 Photoreceptors that provide the perception of color
29 Their axons form the optic nerves
30 Iris, ciliary body, and choroid
31 Region of retina called the "blind spot"

17 _____
18 _____
19 _____
20 _____
21 _____
22 _____
23 _____
24 _____
25 _____
26 _____
27 _____
28 _____
29 _____
30 _____
31 _____

Section integration

A bright flash of light from nearby exploding fireworks blinds Rachel's eyes. The result is a "ghost" image that temporarily remains on her retinas. What might account for the images and their subsequent disappearance?

32 _____

_____

_____

Labeling

Label the structures in this diagram of a sagittal section of the left eye.

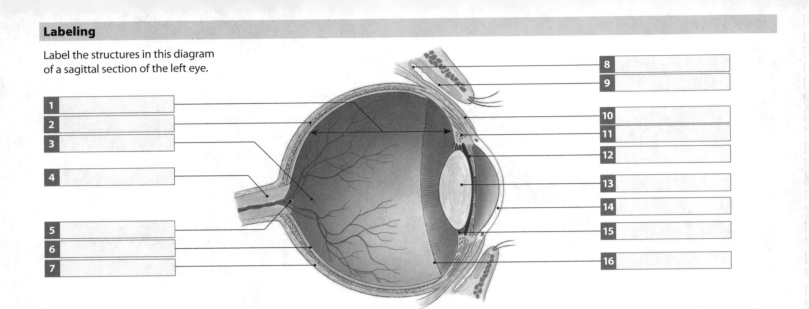

1	
2	
3	
4	
5	
6	
7	
8	
9	
10	
11	
12	
13	
14	
15	
16	

Matching

Match each lettered term with the most closely related description.

a. ganglion cells
b. cones
c. vascular layer
d. rods
e. optic disc
f. posterior chamber
g. crystallins
h. sclera
i. retina
j. occipital lobe
k. palpebrae
l. rhodopsin
m. fovea
n. posterior cavity
o. pupil

17 Visual pigment
18 Eyelids
19 Transparent proteins in the cells of a lens
20 White of the eye
21 Opening surrounded by the iris
22 Inner layer
23 Site of vitreous body
24 Photoreceptors that enable vision in dim light
25 Extends between the iris and the ciliary body and lens
26 Sharpest vision
27 Visual cortex
28 Photoreceptors that provide the perception of color
29 Their axons form the optic nerves
30 Iris, ciliary body, and choroid
31 Region of retina called the "blind spot"

17 _____
18 _____
19 _____
20 _____
21 _____
22 _____
23 _____
24 _____
25 _____
26 _____
27 _____
28 _____
29 _____
30 _____
31 _____

Section integration

A bright flash of light from nearby exploding fireworks blinds Rachel's eyes. The result is a "ghost" image that temporarily remains on her retinas. What might account for the images and their subsequent disappearance?

32 _____

116

Chapter Review Questions

Labeling

Label the structures in this sectional view through the back of the eye.

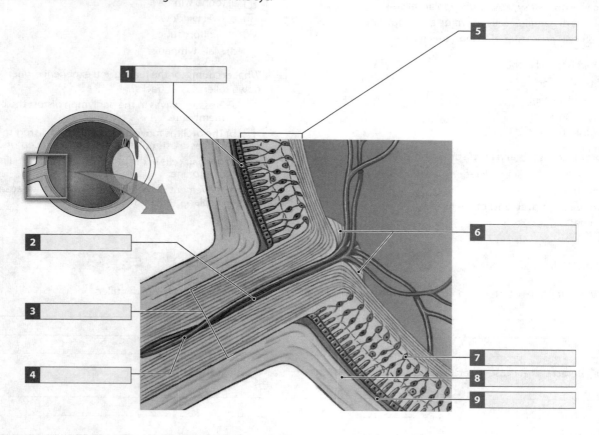

5	
1	
2	
3	
4	
6	
7	
8	
9	

True/False

Indicate whether each statement is true or false.

10 Humans are most sensitive to the sweet taste.

11 The cochlear duct and scala tympani both contain perilymph, and the scala vestibuli contains endolymph.

12 Vibration of the basilar membrane causes vibration of hair cells against the tectorial membrane.

13 The accessory structures of the eye include the fibrous layer, vascular layer, and inner layer.

14 Rods are the photoreceptors that enable vision in dim light.

15 The retinal area of greatest visual acuity is the fovea.

10	_____
11	_____
12	_____
13	_____
14	_____
15	_____

Multiple choice

Select the correct answer from the list provided.

16 A blind spot occurs in the retina where

- ☐ a) the fovea is located.
- ☐ b) ganglion cells synapse with bipolar cells.
- ☐ c) axons of ganglion cells converge at the optic nerve.
- ☐ d) rod cells are clustered to form the macula.

17 The choroid is found in the

- ☐ a) fibrous layer.
- ☐ b) vascular layer.
- ☐ c) inner layer.
- ☐ d) vitreous body.

18 Receptors in the saccule and utricle provide the sensation of

- ☐ a) gravity and linear acceleration.
- ☐ b) hearing.
- ☐ c) rotational movements of the head.
- ☐ d) vibration.

19 The equalization of pressure on either side of the tympanic membrane is achieved by the

- ☐ a) round window.
- ☐ b) oval window.
- ☐ c) auditory tube.
- ☐ d) scala tympani.

20 What accounts for the feeling you experience when you accelerate down rollercoaster tracks?

- ☐ a) Pressure waves in the perilymph distort the basilar membrane.
- ☐ b) The otoliths move horizontally and distort the hair cell processes, stimulating the macular receptors.
- ☐ c) The hair cells in the organ of Corti press against the tectorial membrane.
- ☐ d) Movement of the tympanic membrane causes displacement of the auditory ossicles.

Short answer

21 Identify the four primary taste sensations. Name the two additional taste sensations that have been identified.

_____

_____

_____

22 What is a cataract? What causes a cataract and how is it treated?

_____

_____

_____

23 What is otitis media and what causes it?

_____

_____

_____

Concept map

Use each of the following terms once to fill in the blank boxes to correctly complete the map.

- steroid hormones
- tryptophan derivatives
- glycoproteins
- short polypeptides
- catecholamines
- peptide hormones
- thyroid hormones
- transport proteins
- lipid derivatives
- small proteins
- eicosanoids

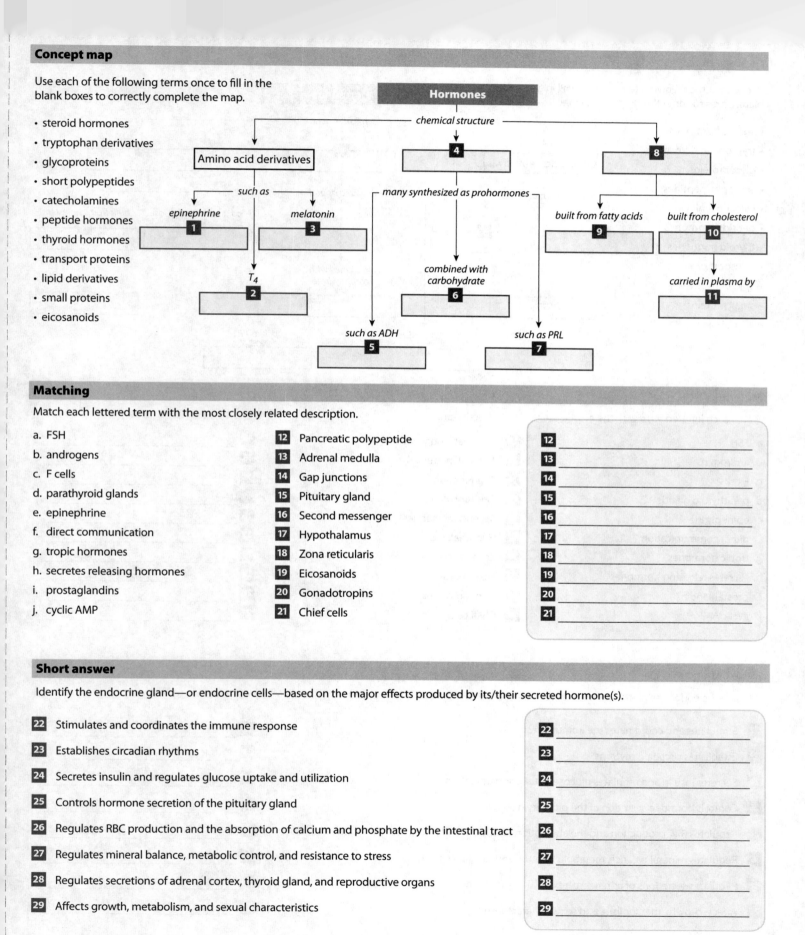

Matching

Match each lettered term with the most closely related description.

a. FSH
b. androgens
c. F cells
d. parathyroid glands
e. epinephrine
f. direct communication
g. tropic hormones
h. secretes releasing hormones
i. prostaglandins
j. cyclic AMP

12	Pancreatic polypeptide	12 _____
13	Adrenal medulla	13 _____
14	Gap junctions	14 _____
15	Pituitary gland	15 _____
16	Second messenger	16 _____
17	Hypothalamus	17 _____
18	Zona reticularis	18 _____
19	Eicosanoids	19 _____
20	Gonadotropins	20 _____
21	Chief cells	21 _____

Short answer

Identify the endocrine gland—or endocrine cells—based on the major effects produced by its/their secreted hormone(s).

22 Stimulates and coordinates the immune response   22 _____

23 Establishes circadian rhythms   23 _____

24 Secretes insulin and regulates glucose uptake and utilization   24 _____

25 Controls hormone secretion of the pituitary gland   25 _____

26 Regulates RBC production and the absorption of calcium and phosphate by the intestinal tract   26 _____

27 Regulates mineral balance, metabolic control, and resistance to stress   27 _____

28 Regulates secretions of adrenal cortex, thyroid gland, and reproductive organs   28 _____

29 Affects growth, metabolism, and sexual characteristics   29 _____

Concept map

Use each of the following terms once to fill in the blank boxes to correctly complete the map.

- steroid hormones
- tryptophan derivatives
- glycoproteins
- short polypeptides
- catecholamines
- peptide hormones
- thyroid hormones
- transport proteins
- lipid derivatives
- small proteins
- eicosanoids

Hormones

chemical structure

Amino acid derivatives | 4 | 8

such as

epinephrine | 1
melatonin | 3

T_4 | 2

many synthesized as prohormones

combined with carbohydrate | 6

such as ADH | 5

such as PRL | 7

built from fatty acids | 9
built from cholesterol | 10

carried in plasma by | 11

Matching

Match each lettered term with the most closely related description.

a. FSH
b. androgens
c. F cells
d. parathyroid glands
e. epinephrine
f. direct communication
g. tropic hormones
h. secretes releasing hormones
i. prostaglandins
j. cyclic AMP

12 Pancreatic polypeptide
13 Adrenal medulla
14 Gap junctions
15 Pituitary gland
16 Second messenger
17 Hypothalamus
18 Zona reticularis
19 Eicosanoids
20 Gonadotropins
21 Chief cells

12 _____
13 _____
14 _____
15 _____
16 _____
17 _____
18 _____
19 _____
20 _____
21 _____

Short answer

Identify the endocrine gland—or endocrine cells—based on the major effects produced by its/their secreted hormone(s).

22 Stimulates and coordinates the immune response

23 Establishes circadian rhythms

24 Secretes insulin and regulates glucose uptake and utilization

25 Controls hormone secretion of the pituitary gland

26 Regulates RBC production and the absorption of calcium and phosphate by the intestinal tract

27 Regulates mineral balance, metabolic control, and resistance to stress

28 Regulates secretions of adrenal cortex, thyroid gland, and reproductive organs

29 Affects growth, metabolism, and sexual characteristics

22 _____
23 _____
24 _____
25 _____
26 _____
27 _____
28 _____
29 _____

120

Labeling

Write the phrases at left in the boxes to complete the diagram of the homeostatic regulation of blood pressure and volume.

- increased fluid loss
- erythropoietin released
- decreased blood pressure
- aldosterone secreted
- suppression of thirst
- decreasing blood pressure and volume
- increasing blood pressure and volume
- renin released
- ADH secreted
- release of natriuretic peptides
- Na$^+$ and H$_2$O loss from kidneys
- increased red blood cell production

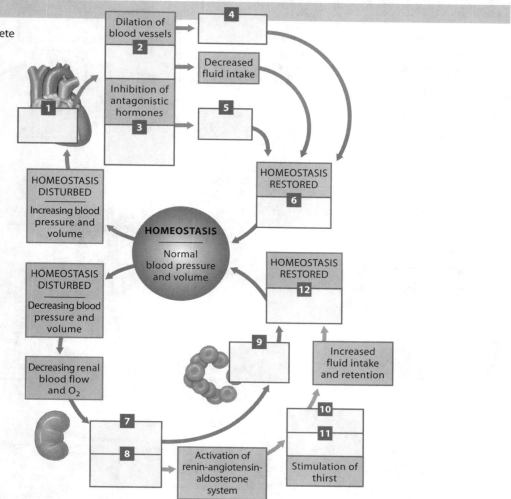

Matching

Match each lettered term with the most closely related description.

a. sympathetic activation
b. decrease blood pressure and volume
c. PTH and calcitonin
d. GH and glucocorticoids
e. increase blood pressure and volume
f. homeostasis threat
g. glucocorticoids
h. PTH and calcitriol
i. gigantism
j. protein synthesis

13	Antagonistic effect	13 _____
14	Resistance phase	14 _____
15	Alarm phase	15 _____
16	Renin and EPO effect	16 _____
17	Growth hormone (GH)	17 _____
18	Additive effect	18 _____
19	Excessive GH in children	19 _____
20	Natriuretic peptides effect	20 _____
21	Stress	21 _____
22	Integrative effect	22 _____

Section integration

Describe, and give an example of, the four possible effects that may occur when a cell receives instructions from two different hormones.

23 _____

_____

Labeling

Write the phrases at left in the boxes to complete the diagram of the homeostatic regulation of blood pressure and volume.

- increased fluid loss
- erythropoietin released
- decreased blood pressure
- aldosterone secreted
- suppression of thirst
- decreasing blood pressure and volume
- increasing blood pressure and volume
- renin released
- ADH secreted
- release of natriuretic peptides
- Na^+ and H_2O loss from kidneys
- increased red blood cell production

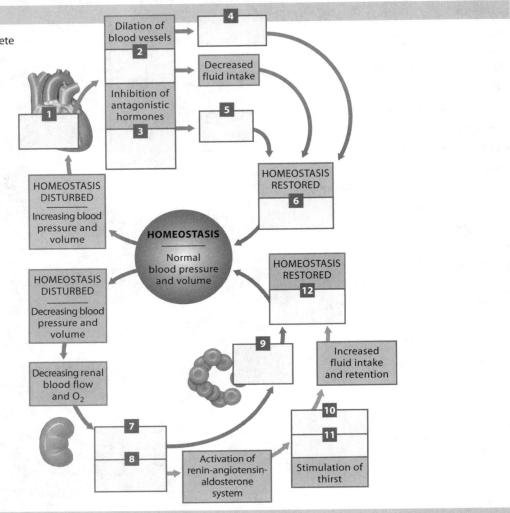

Matching

Match each lettered term with the most closely related description.

a. sympathetic activation

b. decrease blood pressure and volume

c. PTH and calcitonin

d. GH and glucocorticoids

e. increase blood pressure and volume

f. homeostasis threat

g. glucocorticoids

h. PTH and calcitriol

i. gigantism

j. protein synthesis

13	Antagonistic effect
14	Resistance phase
15	Alarm phase
16	Renin and EPO effect
17	Growth hormone (GH)
18	Additive effect
19	Excessive GH in children
20	Natriuretic peptides effect
21	Stress
22	Integrative effect

13 _____
14 _____
15 _____
16 _____
17 _____
18 _____
19 _____
20 _____
21 _____
22 _____

Section integration

Describe, and give an example of, the four possible effects that may occur when a cell receives instructions from two different hormones.

23 _____

_____

Chapter Review Questions

True/False

Indicate whether each statement is true or false.

1 Intercellular communication through extracellular fluid is achieved by paracrine factors.

2 Catecholamines are lipid derivative hormones.

3 Hormones that bind to receptors in the plasma membrane require a second messenger.

4 Rising levels of blood calcium cause the parathyroid glands to secrete PTH.

5 People with Type 2 diabetes must receive insulin daily by injection or through an insulin pump.

1 _____

2 _____

3 _____

4 _____

5 _____

Fill-in

Hypothalamus

Identify the seven regulatory hormones of the hypothalamus.

6 ___ 7 ___ 8 ___ 9 ___ 10 ___ 11 ___ 12 ___

Fill in the boxes with the names of the missing hormones.

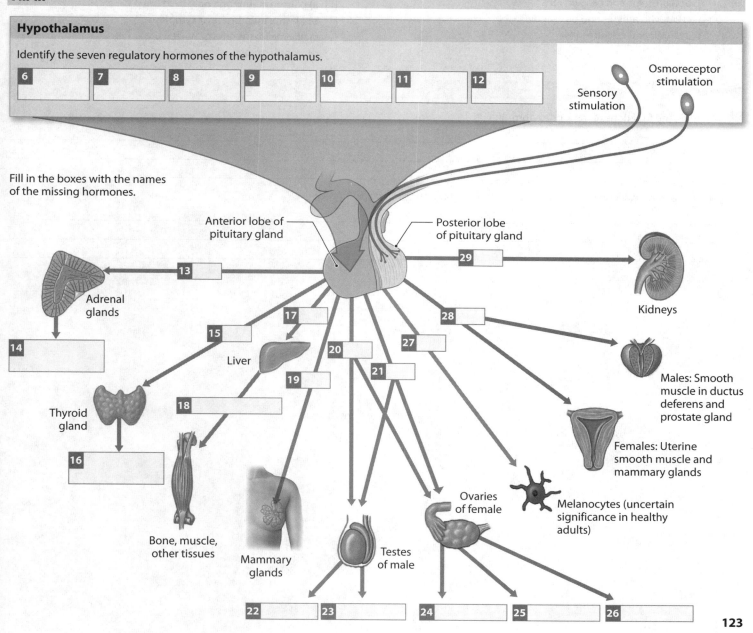

Osmoreceptor stimulation

Sensory stimulation

Anterior lobe of pituitary gland

Posterior lobe of pituitary gland

29 ___

Kidneys

13 ___

Adrenal glands

14 ___

17 ___

28 ___

Males: Smooth muscle in ductus deferens and prostate gland

15 ___

Liver

20 ___

27 ___

Thyroid gland

19 ___

21 ___

Females: Uterine smooth muscle and mammary glands

18 ___

16 ___

Melanocytes (uncertain significance in healthy adults)

Ovaries of female

Bone, muscle, other tissues

Mammary glands

Testes of male

22 ___ 23 ___ 24 ___ 25 ___ 26 ___

Multiple choice

Select the correct answer from the list provided.

30 Secretions from the pancreatic islets are
- a) glucagon from delta cells and insulin from beta cells.
- b) glucagon from alpha cells and insulin from beta cells.
- c) glucagon from beta cells and insulin from alpha cells.
- d) glucagon from beta cells and insulin from delta cells.

31 The pineal gland secretes
- a) corticosteroids.
- b) thyroxine.
- c) melanocyte-stimulating hormone.
- d) melatonin.

32 The two most important second messengers are
- a) cAMP and G proteins.
- b) G proteins and calcium ions.
- c) catecholamines and eicosanoids.
- d) cAMP and calcium ions.

33 FSH production in males supports
- a) physical maturation of developing sperm.
- b) development of muscle size.
- c) the release of androgens.
- d) an increased desire for sexual activity.

34 Which of the following is *not* an effect of thyroid hormones on peripheral tissues?
- a) Increased rates of oxygen consumption and energy
- b) Decreased heart rate
- c) Accelerated turnover of minerals in bone
- d) Increased sensitivity to sympathetic stimulation

35 Steroid hormones bind to receptors in the
- a) plasma membrane only.
- b) plasma membrane or cytoplasm.
- c) plasma membrane or nucleus.
- d) cytoplasm or nucleus.

Short answer

36 What are the functions of the kidney hormones?

_____

_____

_____

37 What effects do calcitonin and parathyroid hormone have on blood calcium levels?

_____

_____

_____

Matching

Use the lettered terms below to fill in the blanks in the diagram.

a. electrolytes
b. globulins
c. 99.9%
d. oxygen transport
e. cell fragments
f. 7%
g. fibrinogen
h. defense mechanisms
i. organic nutrients
j. 92%
k. organic wastes
l. 1%
m. <.1%
n. <.1%
o. albumins

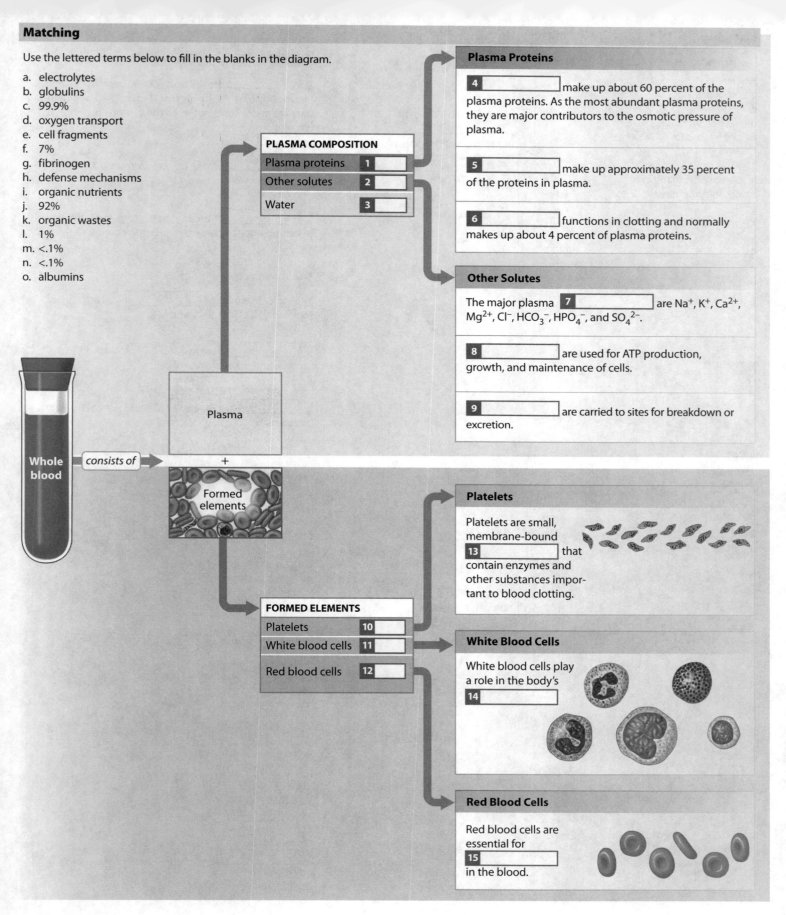

PLASMA COMPOSITION

Plasma proteins	1	
Other solutes	2	
Water	3	

Plasma

+

Formed elements

Whole blood — *consists of* —

Plasma Proteins

4 [_____] make up about 60 percent of the plasma proteins. As the most abundant plasma proteins, they are major contributors to the osmotic pressure of plasma.

5 [_____] make up approximately 35 percent of the proteins in plasma.

6 [_____] functions in clotting and normally makes up about 4 percent of plasma proteins.

Other Solutes

The major plasma **7** [_____] are Na$^+$, K$^+$, Ca^{2+}, Mg^{2+}, Cl$^-$, HCO$_3^-$, HPO$_4^-$, and SO$_4^{2-}$.

8 [_____] are used for ATP production, growth, and maintenance of cells.

9 [_____] are carried to sites for breakdown or excretion.

FORMED ELEMENTS

Platelets	10	
White blood cells	11	
Red blood cells	12	

Platelets

Platelets are small, membrane-bound **13** [_____] that contain enzymes and other substances important to blood clotting.

White Blood Cells

White blood cells play a role in the body's **14** [_____]

Red Blood Cells

Red blood cells are essential for **15** [_____] in the blood.

Matching

Use the lettered terms below to fill in the blanks in the diagram.

a. electrolytes
b. globulins
c. 99.9%
d. oxygen transport
e. cell fragments
f. 7%
g. fibrinogen
h. defense mechanisms
i. organic nutrients
j. 92%
k. organic wastes
l. 1%
m. <.1%
n. <.1%
o. albumins

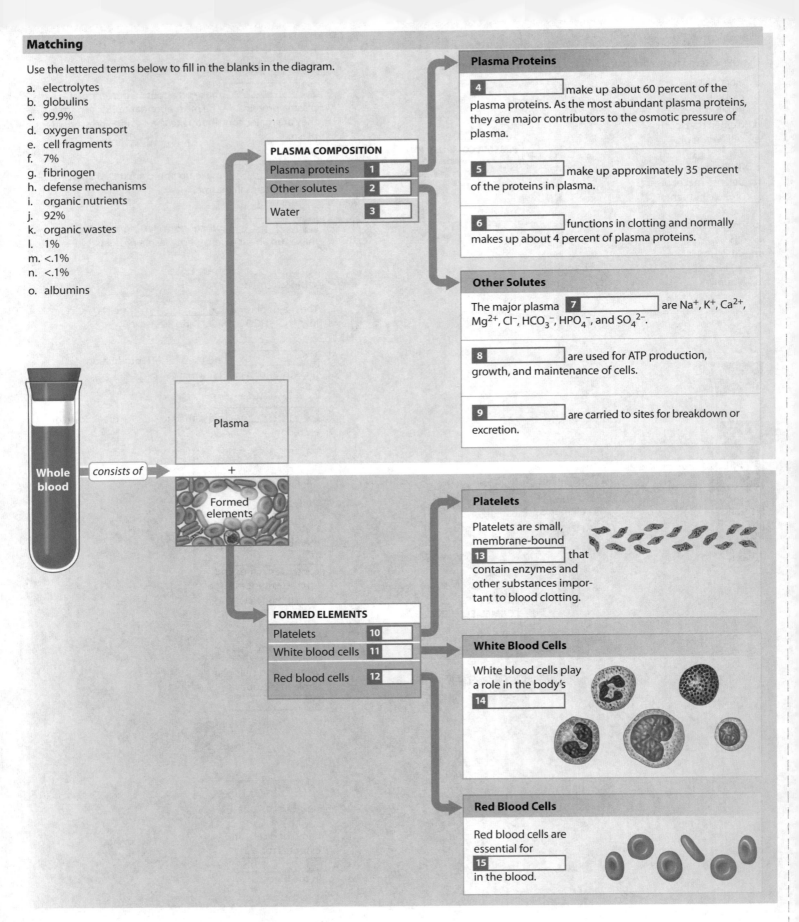

PLASMA COMPOSITION

Plasma proteins	1
Other solutes	2
Water	3

Plasma

Whole blood — consists of →

+

Formed elements

FORMED ELEMENTS

Platelets	10
White blood cells	11
Red blood cells	12

Plasma Proteins

4 [_____] make up about 60 percent of the plasma proteins. As the most abundant plasma proteins, they are major contributors to the osmotic pressure of plasma.

5 [_____] make up approximately 35 percent of the proteins in plasma.

6 [_____] functions in clotting and normally makes up about 4 percent of plasma proteins.

Other Solutes

The major plasma **7** [_____] are Na^+, K^+, Ca^{2+}, Mg^{2+}, Cl^-, HCO_3^-, HPO_4^-, and SO_4^{2-}.

8 [_____] are used for ATP production, growth, and maintenance of cells.

9 [_____] are carried to sites for breakdown or excretion.

Platelets

Platelets are small, membrane-bound **13** [_____] that contain enzymes and other substances important to blood clotting.

White Blood Cells

White blood cells play a role in the body's **14** [_____]

Red Blood Cells

Red blood cells are essential for **15** [_____] in the blood.

Concept map

Use each of the following terms once to fill in
the blank boxes to correctly complete the map.

- globulins
- electrolytes, glucose, urea
- proteins
- albumins
- leukocytes
- fibrinogen
- solutes
- basophils
- erythrocytes
- formed elements
- plasma
- eosinophils
- lymphocytes
- water
- platelets
- monocytes
- neutrophils

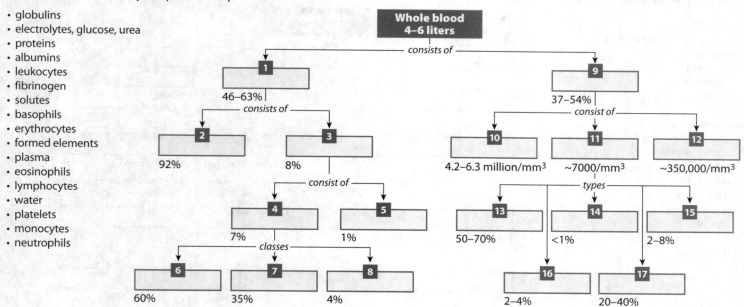

Matching

Match each lettered description with the most closely related term.

a. matrix	**18** Myeloid tissue	**18** _____
b. transport protein	**19** Anucleated	**19** _____
c. jaundice	**20** Plasma	**20** _____
d. venipuncture	**21** Macrophages	**21** _____
e. red bone marrow	**22** Globulin	**22** _____
f. mature RBCs	**23** Agglutination	**23** _____
g. pigment complex	**24** Specific immunity	**24** _____
h. platelets	**25** Bilirubin	**25** _____
i. erythropoietin	**26** Median cubital vein	**26** _____
j. cross-reaction	**27** Heme	**27** _____
k. monocytes	**28** Hormone	**28** _____
l. lymphocytes	**29** Blood clotting	**29** _____

Section integration

Why are mature red blood cells in humans incapable of protein synthesis and mitosis?

30 _____

_____

_____

Concept map

Use each of the following terms once to fill in the blank boxes to correctly complete the map.

- globulins
- electrolytes, glucose, urea
- proteins
- albumins
- leukocytes
- fibrinogen
- solutes
- basophils
- erythrocytes
- formed elements
- plasma
- eosinophils
- lymphocytes
- water
- platelets
- monocytes
- neutrophils

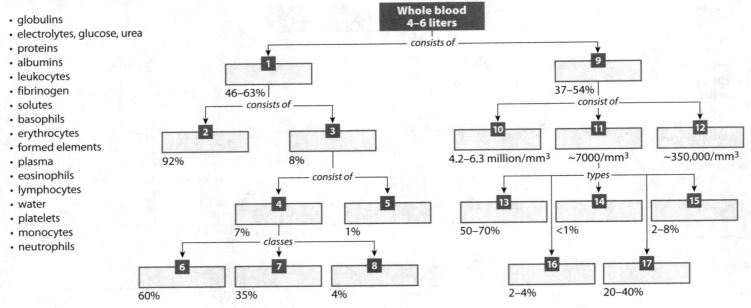

Matching

Match each lettered description with the most closely related term.

a. matrix
b. transport protein
c. jaundice
d. venipuncture
e. red bone marrow
f. mature RBCs
g. pigment complex
h. platelets
i. erythropoietin
j. cross-reaction
k. monocytes
l. lymphocytes

18	Myeloid tissue	18 _____
19	Anucleated	19 _____
20	Plasma	20 _____
21	Macrophages	21 _____
22	Globulin	22 _____
23	Agglutination	23 _____
24	Specific immunity	24 _____
25	Bilirubin	25 _____
26	Median cubital vein	26 _____
27	Heme	27 _____
28	Hormone	28 _____
29	Blood clotting	29 _____

Section integration

Why are mature red blood cells in humans incapable of protein synthesis and mitosis?

30 _____

_____

_____

Chapter Review Questions

Labeling

Label the blood cells shown here.

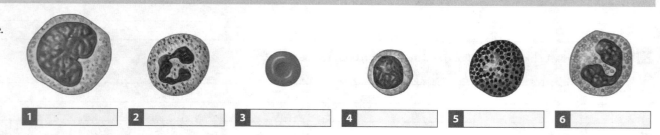

| 1 | 2 | 3 | 4 | 5 | 6 |

True/False

Indicate whether each statement is true or false.

7 Globulins make up 60 percent of the plasma proteins.

8 Monocytes enter damaged tissues and release histamines that promote inflammation.

9 Red blood cells have an average life span of 120 days.

10 The first phase of hemostasis is the coagulation phase.

11 Neutrophils are the most abundant white blood cells.

7 _____

8 _____

9 _____

10 _____

11 _____

Multiple choice

Select the correct answer from the list provided.

12 Plasma _____ percentage of the whole blood volume; formed elements _____ percentage of whole blood volume.
- [ ] a) 55, 45
- [ ] b) 45, 55
- [ ] c) 92, 8
- [ ] d) 63, 37

13 A hemoglobin molecule is composed of
- [ ] a) two protein chains and two heme units.
- [ ] b) four protein chains and two heme units.
- [ ] c) four protein chains and four heme units.
- [ ] d) one protein chain and one heme unit.

14 The correct order of erythrocyte formation is
- [ ] a) hematopoietic stem cell, myeloid stem cell, progenitor cell, proerythroblast, erythroblast stages, reticulocyte, erythrocyte.
- [ ] b) hematopoietic stem cell, progenitor cell, myeloid stem cell, proerythroblast, reticulocyte, erythroblast stages, erythrocyte.
- [ ] c) hematopoietic stem cell, myeloid stem cell, progenitor cell, reticulocyte, proerythroblast, erythroblast stages, erythrocyte.
- [ ] d) myeloid stem cell, hematopoietic stem cell, progenitor cell, proerythroblast, reticulocyte, erythroblast stages, erythrocyte.

15 Megakaryocytes shed cytoplasm in small, membrane-enclosed packets that enter the bloodstream as
- [ ] a) neutrophils.
- [ ] b) lymphocytes.
- [ ] c) monocytes.
- [ ] d) platelets.

16 Which of the following blood types is the "universal donor"?
- [ ] a) O^+
- [ ] b) O^-
- [ ] c) AB^+
- [ ] d) AB^-

17 When an RBC is engulfed by a macrophage, the hemoglobin heme units are stripped of their iron and converted to
- [ ] a) bilirubin.
- [ ] b) biliverdin.
- [ ] c) urobilins.
- [ ] d) stercobilins.

18 The percentage of formed elements in a sample of whole blood is called
- [ ] a) hemoglobinuria.
- [ ] b) hematocrit.
- [ ] c) hematuria.
- [ ] d) oxyhemoglobin.

Short answer

19 Describe the various types of leukemias.

20 What is the role of blood in stabilizing and maintaining body temperature?

21 Identify the RBC surface antigens and plasma antibodies for blood types A, B, AB, and O.

Labeling

Label the blood vessels and their components in the images below.

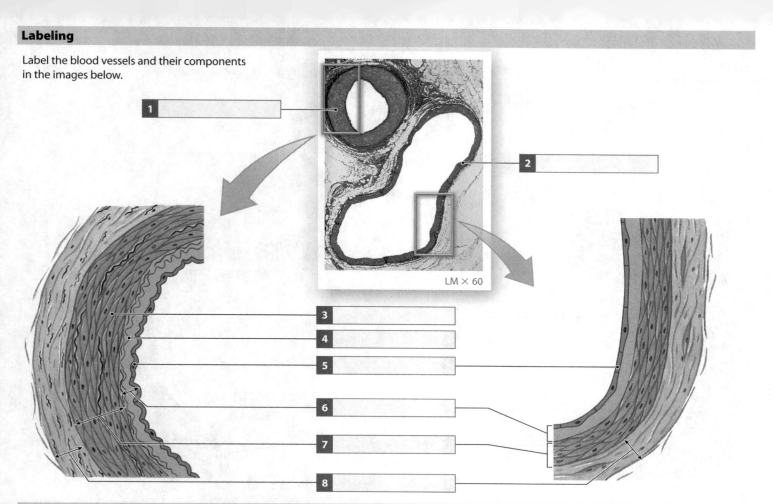

1 _____

2 _____

LM × 60

3 _____

4 _____

5 _____

6 _____

7 _____

8 _____

Matching

Match each lettered term with the most closely related description.

a. pulmonary circuit
b. vein
c. exchange vessels
d. continuous capillary
e. systemic circuit
f. right atrium
g. venous valves
h. fenestrated capillaries
i. artery
j. anastomosis
k. sinusoids
l. tunica media

9   Left ventricle pumps blood into this
10   Relatively thick wall
11   Joining of blood vessels
12   Present only in veins
13   Blood to and from the lungs
14   Present in liver, bone marrow, and spleen
15   Relatively thin wall
16   Contain pores
17   Smooth muscle tissue
18   Capillaries
19   Complete endothelial lining
20   Receives blood from systemic circuit

9 _____
10 _____
11 _____
12 _____
13 _____
14 _____
15 _____
16 _____
17 _____
18 _____
19 _____
20 _____

Section integration

What is the function of precapillary sphincters, and what role would you expect them to play during exercise and in cold temperatures?

21 _____

Labeling

Label the blood vessels and their components in the images below.

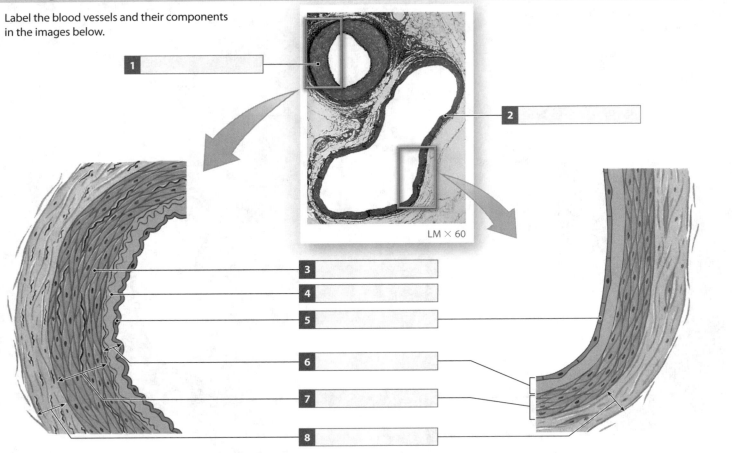

1 _____

2 _____

LM × 60

3 _____

4 _____

5 _____

6 _____

7 _____

8 _____

Matching

Match each lettered term with the most closely related description.

a. pulmonary circuit

b. vein

c. exchange vessels

d. continuous capillary

e. systemic circuit

f. right atrium

g. venous valves

h. fenestrated capillaries

i. artery

j. anastomosis

k. sinusoids

l. tunica media

9　Left ventricle pumps blood into this

10　Relatively thick wall

11　Joining of blood vessels

12　Present only in veins

13　Blood to and from the lungs

14　Present in liver, bone marrow, and spleen

15　Relatively thin wall

16　Contain pores

17　Smooth muscle tissue

18　Capillaries

19　Complete endothelial lining

20　Receives blood from systemic circuit

9 _____

10 _____

11 _____

12 _____

13 _____

14 _____

15 _____

16 _____

17 _____

18 _____

19 _____

20 _____

Section integration

What is the function of precapillary sphincters, and what role would you expect them to play during exercise and in cold temperatures?

21 _____

Labeling

Label the major arteries in the diagram at right.

1 _____
2 _____
3 _____
4 _____
5 _____
6 _____
7 _____
8 _____
9 _____
10 _____
11 _____
12 _____
13 _____
14 _____

Label the major veins in the diagram below.

15 _____
16 _____
17 _____
18 _____
19 _____
20 _____
21 _____
22 _____
23 _____
24 _____
25 _____
26 _____
27 _____
28 _____

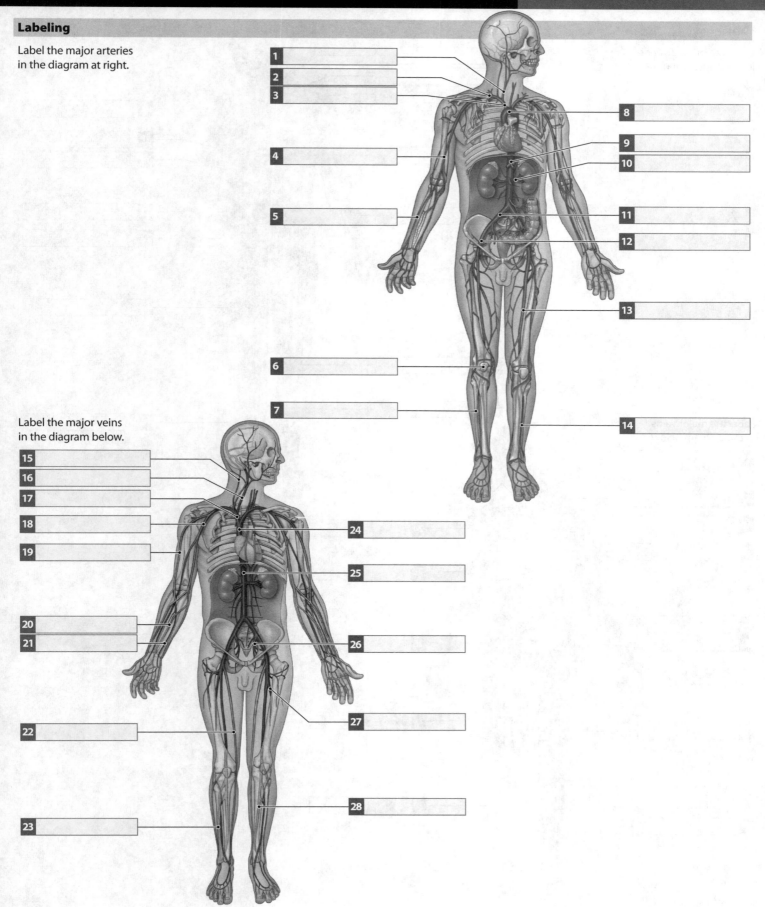

Labeling

Label the major arteries in the diagram at right.

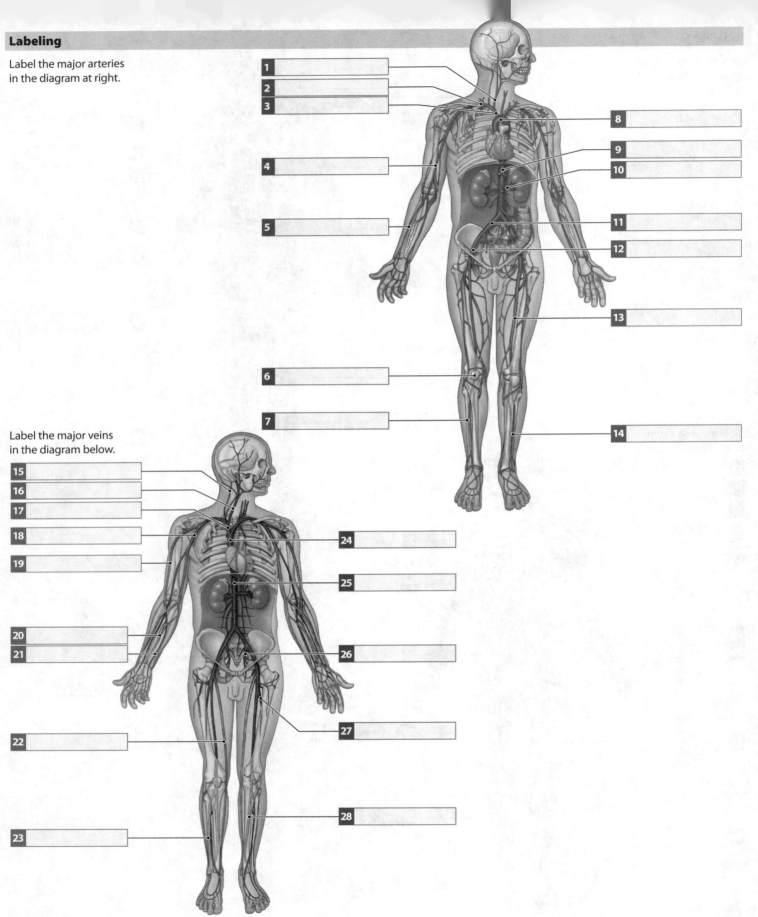

1

2

3

4

5

6

7

8

9

10

11

12

13

14

Label the major veins in the diagram below.

15

16

17

18

19

20

21

22

23

24

25

26

27

28

Chapter Review Questions

Labeling

Label the arteries of the brain shown in the image below.

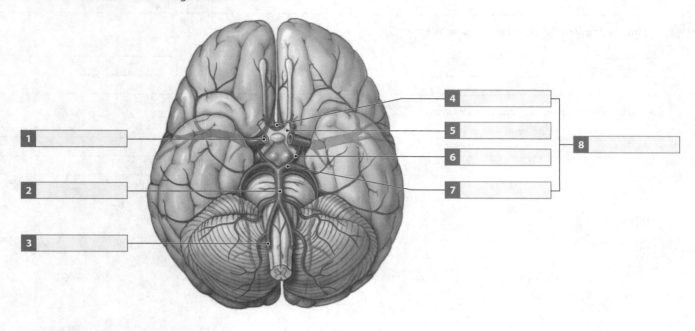

Multiple choice

Select the correct answer from the list provided.

9 The heart pumps blood into the systemic circuit from the

- a) right atrium.
- b) right ventricle.
- c) left atrium.
- d) left ventricle.

10 The blood vessel layer containing smooth muscle fibers allowing for the processes of vasoconstriction and vasodilation is the

- a) tunica intima.
- b) tunica media.
- c) tunica adventitia.
- d) tunica externa.

11 Capillaries containing pores that permit the passage of large molecules are

- a) continous capillaries.
- b) precapillary sphincters.
- c) collaterals.
- d) fenestrated capillaries.

12 Most of the body's total blood volume is distributed within the

- a) pulmonary circuit.
- b) systemic arterial system.
- c) systemic venous system.
- d) systemic capillaries.

13 The process of generating blood vessels from pre-existing vessels is called

- a) angiogenesis.
- b) vasculogenesis.
- c) fenestration.
- d) arteriosus.

14 Which of the following is the correct combination of celiac trunk branches?

- a) common hepatic artery, superior mesenteric artery, inferior mesenteric artery
- b) common hepatic artery, splenic artery, superior mesenteric artery
- c) common hepatic artery, left gastric artery, phrenic artery
- d) common hepatic artery, left gastric artery, splenic artery

15 The vein that drains the venous sinuses of the brain is the

- a) internal jugular vein.
- b) external jugular vein.
- c) vertebral vein.
- d) great cerebral vein.

16 The two branches from the brachiocephalic trunk are the

- a) left subclavian and left common carotid arteries.
- b) right subclavian and right common carotid arteries.
- c) left subclavian and left common carotid veins.
- d) right subclavian and right common carotid veins.

Short answer

17 The brachiocephalic trunk branches from the right side of the aortic arch. Why is there no such vessel on the left side?

18 List the distribution of the body's total blood volume.

19 Describe the function of the hepatic portal system.

Labeling

Label each of the structures in this figure.

1	
2	
3	
4	
5	
6	
7	
8	
9	
10	
11	
12	
13	
14	
15	
16	
17	
18	
19	
20	
21	
22	
23	
24	

Matching

Match each lettered term with the most closely related description.

a. fossa ovalis

b. intercalated discs

c. serous membrane

d. tricuspid valve

e. aortic valve

f. endocardium

g. aorta

h. myocardium

i. mitral valve

j. coronary sinus

25 Blood to systemic arteries

26 Muscular wall of heart

27 Carries blood from coronary veins to right atrium

28 Depression in interatrial septum

29 Right atrioventricular valve

30 Alternate name for bicuspid valve

31 Cardiac muscle fiber connections

32 Pericardium

33 Inner surface of heart

34 Semilunar valve

25 _____

26 _____

27 _____

28 _____

29 _____

30 _____

31 _____

32 _____

33 _____

34 _____

Short answer

Beginning with the right atrium, list in order the heart chambers and valves through which (a) deoxygenated blood and (b) oxygenated blood flows.

35 _____

_____

Labeling

Label each of the structures in this figure.

1

2

3

4

5

6

7

8

9

10

11

12

13

14

15

16

17

18

19

20

21

22

23

24

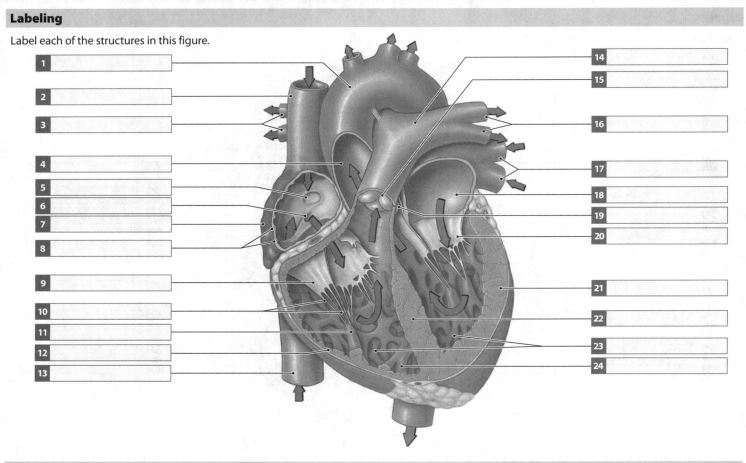

Matching

Match each lettered term with the most closely related description.

a. fossa ovalis

b. intercalated discs

c. serous membrane

d. tricuspid valve

e. aortic valve

f. endocardium

g. aorta

h. myocardium

i. mitral valve

j. coronary sinus

25 Blood to systemic arteries

26 Muscular wall of heart

27 Carries blood from coronary veins to right atrium

28 Depression in interatrial septum

29 Right atrioventricular valve

30 Alternate name for bicuspid valve

31 Cardiac muscle fiber connections

32 Pericardium

33 Inner surface of heart

34 Semilunar valve

25

26

27

28

29

30

31

32

33

34

Short answer

Beginning with the right atrium, list in order the heart chambers and valves through which
(a) deoxygenated blood and (b) oxygenated blood flows.

35

Matching

Match each lettered term with the most closely related description.

a. P wave

b. cardiac output

c. automaticity

d. "lubb" sound

e. "dupp" sound

f. sympathetic neurons

g. stroke volume

h. tachycardia

i. bradycardia

j. parasympathetic neurons

1	AV valves close
2	Self-stimulated cardiac muscle contractions
3	Atrial depolarization
4	Amount of blood ejected by ventricle during a single beat
5	HR × SV
6	Decrease the heart rate
7	Term for slower-than-normal HR
8	Increase the heart rate
9	Semilunar valve closes
10	Term for faster-than-normal HR

1 _____

2 _____

3 _____

4 _____

5 _____

6 _____

7 _____

8 _____

9 _____

10 _____

Short answer

Refer to the accompanying graph of the cardiac cycle to answer the questions below.

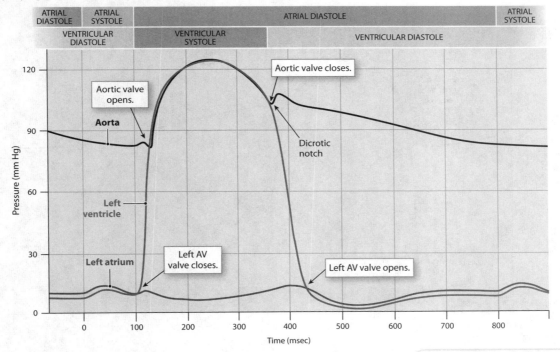

11 What event occurs when the pressure in the left ventricle rises above that in the left atrium?

11 _____

12 During ventricular systole, the blood volume in the **atria** is (increasing or decreasing)?

12 _____

13 During ventricular systole, the volume in the **ventricles** is (increasing or decreasing)?

13 _____

14 During most of ventricular diastole, the pressure in the left ventricle is (greater than, the same as, or less than) the pressure in the left atrium.

14 _____

15 What event occurs when the pressure within the left ventricle becomes greater than the pressure within the aorta?

15 _____

16 During isovolumetric contraction, where is pressure the highest?

16 _____

17 During what part of the cardiac cycle is blood pressure highest in the large systemic arteries?

17 _____

Matching

Match each lettered term with the most closely related description.

a. P wave

b. cardiac output

c. automaticity

d. "lubb" sound

e. "dupp" sound

f. sympathetic neurons

g. stroke volume

h. tachycardia

i. bradycardia

j. parasympathetic neurons

1 AV valves close

2 Self-stimulated cardiac muscle contractions

3 Atrial depolarization

4 Amount of blood ejected by ventricle during a single beat

5 HR × SV

6 Decrease the heart rate

7 Term for slower-than-normal HR

8 Increase the heart rate

9 Semilunar valve closes

10 Term for faster-than-normal HR

1 _____

2 _____

3 _____

4 _____

5 _____

6 _____

7 _____

8 _____

9 _____

10 _____

Short answer

Refer to the accompanying graph of the cardiac cycle to answer the questions below.

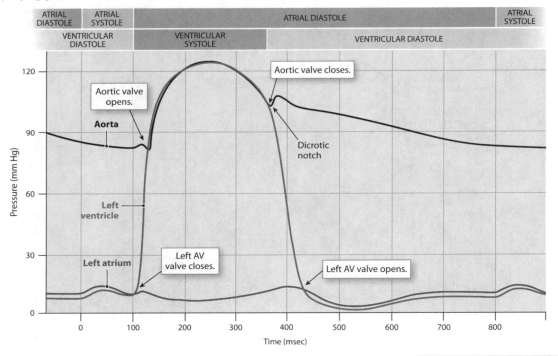

11 What event occurs when the pressure in the left ventricle rises above that in the left atrium?

12 During ventricular systole, the blood volume in the **atria** is (increasing or decreasing)?

13 During ventricular systole, the volume in the **ventricles** is (increasing or decreasing)?

14 During most of ventricular diastole, the pressure in the left ventricle is (greater than, the same as, or less than) the pressure in the left atrium.

15 What event occurs when the pressure within the left ventricle becomes greater than the pressure within the aorta?

16 During isovolumetric contraction, where is pressure the highest?

17 During what part of the cardiac cycle is blood pressure highest in the large systemic arteries?

11 _____

12 _____

13 _____

14 _____

15 _____

16 _____

17 _____

Matching

Match each lettered term with the most closely related description.

a. autoregulation

b. venous return

c. local vasodilators

d. natriuretic peptides

e. chemoreceptors

f. baroreceptors

g. turbulence

h. net hydrostatic pressure

i. medulla oblongata

j. edema

k. viscosity

l. osmotic pressure

1 Detect changes in pressure

2 Vasomotor center

3 Aided by thoracic pressure changes due to breathing

4 Causes immediate, local homeostatic responses

5 Decreased tissue O_2 and increased CO_2

6 Carotid bodies

7 Forces water into a capillary

8 Opposite of smooth blood flow

9 Resistance to flow

10 Forces water out of a capillary

11 Peripheral vasodilation

12 Excess interstitial fluid accumulation

1 _____
2 _____
3 _____
4 _____
5 _____
6 _____
7 _____
8 _____
9 _____
10 _____
11 _____
12 _____

Match each lettered item with the appropriate numbered blank box in the diagram below.

a. increased cardiac output and peripheral vasoconstriction

b. aldosterone secreted

c. increased blood pressure

d. blood pressure and volume decrease

e. thirst stimulated

f. increased blood volume

g. blood pressure and volume increase

h. antidiuretic hormone released

i. increased red blood cell formation

j. widepread vasoconstriction

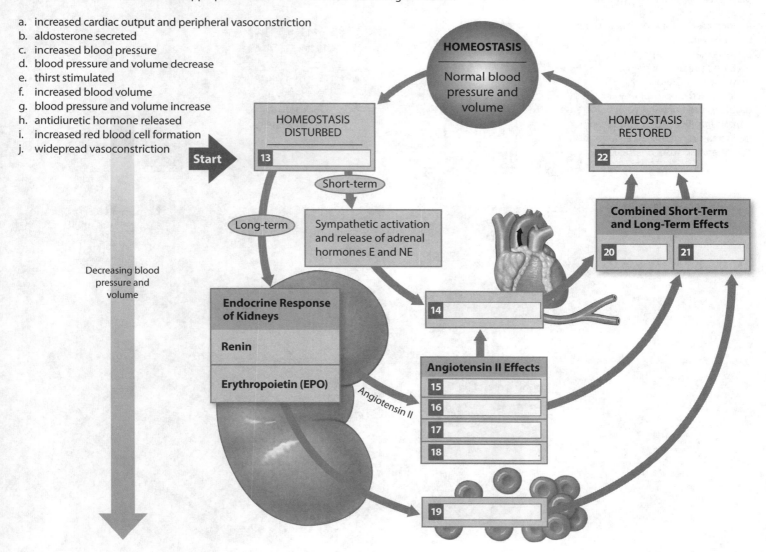

Matching

Match each lettered term with the most closely related description.

a. autoregulation
b. venous return
c. local vasodilators
d. natriuretic peptides
e. chemoreceptors
f. baroreceptors
g. turbulence
h. net hydrostatic pressure
i. medulla oblongata
j. edema
k. viscosity
l. osmotic pressure

1	Detect changes in pressure
2	Vasomotor center
3	Aided by thoracic pressure changes due to breathing
4	Causes immediate, local homeostatic responses
5	Decreased tissue O_2 and increased CO_2
6	Carotid bodies
7	Forces water into a capillary
8	Opposite of smooth blood flow
9	Resistance to flow
10	Forces water out of a capillary
11	Peripheral vasodilation
12	Excess interstitial fluid accumulation

1	_____
2	_____
3	_____
4	_____
5	_____
6	_____
7	_____
8	_____
9	_____
10	_____
11	_____
12	_____

Match each lettered item with the appropriate numbered blank box in the diagram below.

a. increased cardiac output and peripheral vasoconstriction
b. aldosterone secreted
c. increased blood pressure
d. blood pressure and volume decrease
e. thirst stimulated
f. increased blood volume
g. blood pressure and volume increase
h. antidiuretic hormone released
i. increased red blood cell formation
j. widepread vasoconstriction

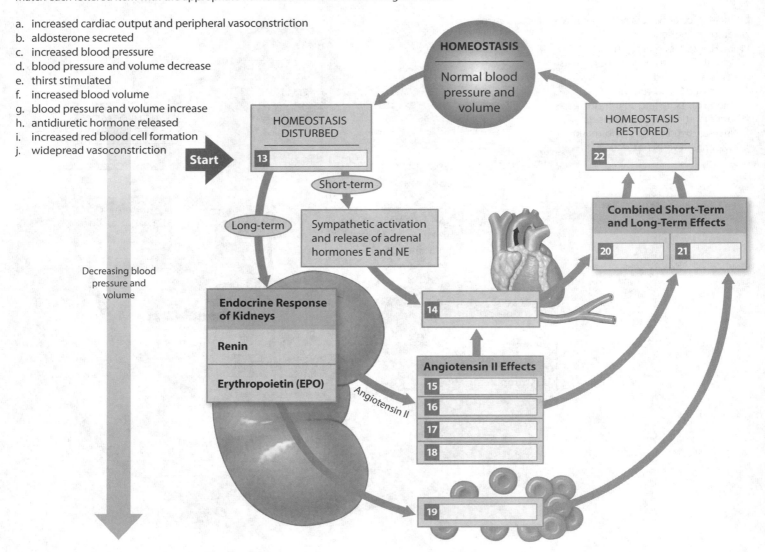

Chapter Review Questions

True/False

Indicate whether each statement is true or false.

1. The S_1 or "lubb" sound of the heart is produced by the AV valves closing.

2. The T wave of an electrocardiogram represents repolarization of the atria.

3. The circumflex artery supplies blood to the surface of the right ventricle.

4. Isovolumetric contraction is the first phase of ventricular systole, when pressures close the AV valves, but are not high enough to open the semilunar valves.

5. Tachycardia is a faster-than-normal heart rate, usually above 100 bpm.

1. _____

2. _____

3. _____

4. _____

5. _____

Multiple choice

Select the correct answer from the list provided.

6. Cardiac output (CO) is calculated by which of the following formulas?
   - a) CO = HR × ESV
   - b) CO = HR × EDV
   - c) CO = HR × SV
   - d) CO = HR × MAP

7. During diastole, a chamber of the heart
   - a) relaxes and fills with blood.
   - b) contracts and pushes blood into the adjacent chamber.
   - c) experiences a sharp increase in pressure.
   - d) reaches a pressure of approximately 120 mm Hg.

8. Which of the following is longer?
   - a) the refractory period of a skeletal muscle fiber
   - b) the refractory period of a cardiac muscle cell
   - c) the action potential of a skeletal muscle fiber
   - d) the contraction time of a skeletal muscle fiber

9. If the papillary muscles fail to contract
   - a) the AV valves will not open.
   - b) the semilunar valves will not open.
   - c) the AV valves will not close properly.
   - d) the semilunar valves will not close properly.

10. The right atrium does *not* receive blood from the
    - a) inferior vena cava.
    - b) superior vena cava.
    - c) coronary sinus.
    - d) circumflex artery.

11. Which of the following is a fibrous remnant of a fetal connection between the aorta and pulmonary trunk?
    - a) fossa ovalis
    - b) ligamentum arteriosum
    - c) chordae tendineae
    - d) trabeculae carneae

12. The Frank-Starling law of the heart states that
    - a) the greater the EDV, the greater the stroke volume.
    - b) the greater the ESV, the greater the stroke volume.
    - c) the greater the EDV, the lesser the stroke volume.
    - d) the lesser the ESV, the lesser the stroke volume.

13. Which of the following homeostatic disturbances will cause a chemoreceptor reflex response?
    - a) increased pH in blood
    - b) increased CO_2 in blood
    - c) increased O_2 in blood
    - d) increased O_2 in CSF

14. Which of the following organs receives an unchanging flow of blood as exercise intensity increases?
    - a) brain
    - b) kidney
    - c) skin
    - d) skeletal muscles

15. Abnormal stretch of the right atrium due to excessive blood volume triggers cardiac muscle cells to release
    - a) brain natriuretic peptide (BNP).
    - b) erythropoietin (EPO).
    - c) angiotensin-converting enzyme (ACE).
    - d) atrial natriuretic peptide (ANP).

Short answer

16 What role do the chordae tendineae and papillary muscles play in the normal function of the AV valves?

17 Trace the normal pathway of an electrical impulse through the conducting system of the heart.

18 Describe the three distinct layers that make up the heart wall.

19 What effects do sympathetic and parasympathetic stimulation have on the heart?

20 What are the sources and significance of the four heart sounds?

Label the structures of the lymphatic system
in the accompanying figure.

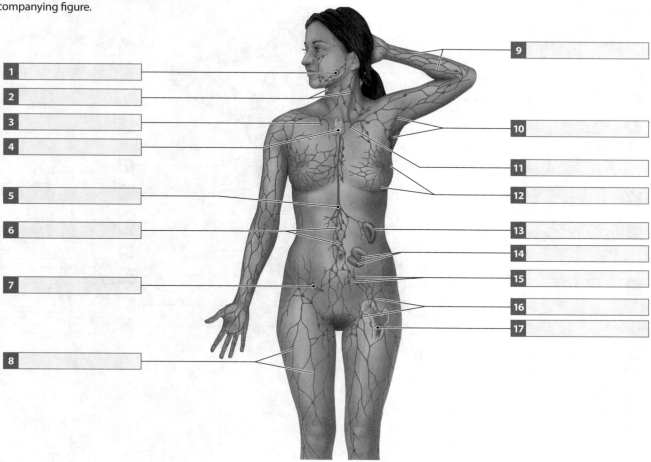

1

2

3

4

5

6

7

8

9

10

11

12

13

14

15

16

17

Match each lettered term with the most closely related description.

a. B cells

b. spleen

c. lymphatic capillaries

d. cytotoxic T cells

e. epithelial cells

f. tonsils

g. lymphopoiesis

h. thymic corpuscles

i. lymphoid organs

j. helper T cells and suppressor T cells

k. afferent lymphatics

l. right subclavian vein

m. lymph nodes

18 Beginning of lymphatic system

19 Thymus medullary cells

20 Receives lymph from right lymphatic duct

21 Thymus, spleen, and lymph nodes

22 Smallest lymphoid organs

23 Regulate and coordinate the immune response

24 Largest mass of lymphoid tissue in body

25 Maintains blood–thymus barrier

26 Occurs in red bone marrow, thymus, and lymphoid tissues

27 Cell-mediated immunity

28 Lymphoid nodules in walls of pharynx

29 Antibody-mediated immunity

30 Carry lymph to lymph nodes

18 _____

19 _____

20 _____

21 _____

22 _____

23 _____

24 _____

25 _____

26 _____

27 _____

28 _____

29 _____

30 _____

Labeling

Label the structures of the lymphatic system in the accompanying figure.

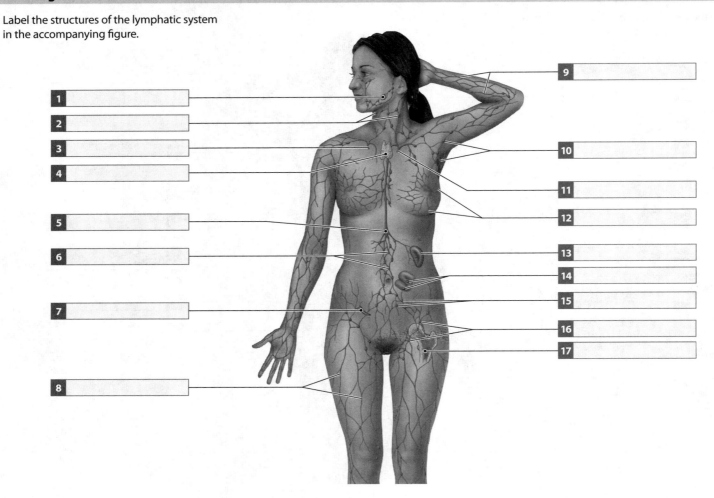

1	
2	
3	
4	
5	
6	
7	
8	

9	
10	
11	
12	
13	
14	
15	
16	
17	

Matching

Match each lettered term with the most closely related description.

a. B cells

b. spleen

c. lymphatic capillaries

d. cytotoxic T cells

e. epithelial cells

f. tonsils

g. lymphopoiesis

h. thymic corpuscles

i. lymphoid organs

j. helper T cells and suppressor T cells

k. afferent lymphatics

l. right subclavian vein

m. lymph nodes

18	Beginning of lymphatic system	18	_____
19	Thymus medullary cells	19	_____
20	Receives lymph from right lymphatic duct	20	_____
21	Thymus, spleen, and lymph nodes	21	_____
22	Smallest lymphoid organs	22	_____
23	Regulate and coordinate the immune response	23	_____
24	Largest mass of lymphoid tissue in body	24	_____
25	Maintains blood–thymus barrier	25	_____
26	Occurs in red bone marrow, thymus, and lymphoid tissues	26	_____
27	Cell-mediated immunity	27	_____
28	Lymphoid nodules in walls of pharynx	28	_____
29	Antibody-mediated immunity	29	_____
30	Carry lymph to lymph nodes	30	_____

Labeling

Identify the type of innate immunity (nonspecific defense) described below.

1 keep hazardous organisms and materials outside the body. For example, a mosquito that lands on your head may be unable to reach the surface of the scalp if you have a full head of hair.	
2 are cells that engulf pathogens and cell debris. Examples are the macrophages of peripheral tissues and the eosinophils and neutrophils of blood.	
3 is the destruction of abnormal cells by NK cells in peripheral tissues.	Destruction of abnormal cells
4 are chemical messengers that coordinate the defenses against viral infections.	
5 is a system of circulating proteins that assists antibodies in the destruction of pathogens.	
6 is a localized, tissue-level response that tends to limit the spread of an injury or infection.	Inflammation
7 is an elevation of body temperature that accelerates tissue metabolism and the activity of defenses.	

1 _____

2 _____

3 _____

4 _____

5 _____

6 _____

7 _____

Multiple choice

Select the correct answer from the list provided.

8 A physical barrier such as the skin provides a nonspecific body defense due to its makeup, which includes

- a) multiple layers.
- b) a coating of keratinized cells.
- c) a network of desmosomes locking adjacent cells together.
- d) all of these.

9 NK cells sensitive to the presence of abnormal plasma membranes are primarily involved in

- a) defenses against specific threats.
- b) phagocytic activity for defense.
- c) complex, time-consuming defense mechanisms.
- d) immune surveillance.

10 The nonspecific defense that breaks down cells, attracts phagocytes, and stimulates inflammation is

- a) the inflammatory response.
- b) the action of interferons.
- c) the complement system.
- d) immune surveillance.

11 The protein(s) that interfere with the replication of viruses is (are)

- a) complement proteins.
- b) heparin.
- c) pyrogens.
- d) interferons.

12 Circulating proteins that reset the thermostat in the hypothalamus, causing a rise in body temperature, are called

- a) pyrogens.
- b) interferons.
- c) lysosomes.
- d) complement proteins.

13 The "first line of cellular defense" against pathogenic invasion is

- a) phagocytes.
- b) mucus.
- c) hair.
- d) interferon.

Short answer

We usually associate a fever with illness or disease. How can a fever be beneficial?

14 _____

Labeling

Identify the type of innate immunity (nonspecific defense) described below.

1 keep hazardous organisms and materials outside the body. For example, a mosquito that lands on your head may be unable to reach the surface of the scalp if you have a full head of hair.	
2 are cells that engulf pathogens and cell debris. Examples are the macrophages of peripheral tissues and the eosinophils and neutrophils of blood.	
3 is the destruction of abnormal cells by NK cells in peripheral tissues.	Destruction of abnormal cells
4 are chemical messengers that coordinate the defenses against viral infections.	
5 is a system of circulating proteins that assists antibodies in the destruction of pathogens.	
6 is a localized, tissue-level response that tends to limit the spread of an injury or infection.	Inflammation
7 is an elevation of body temperature that accelerates tissue metabolism and the activity of defenses.	

1 _____

2 _____

3 _____

4 _____

5 _____

6 _____

7 _____

Multiple choice

Select the correct answer from the list provided.

8 A physical barrier such as the skin provides a nonspecific body defense due to its makeup, which includes

- [ ] a) multiple layers.
- [ ] b) a coating of keratinized cells.
- [ ] c) a network of desmosomes locking adjacent cells together.
- [ ] d) all of these.

9 NK cells sensitive to the presence of abnormal plasma membranes are primarily involved in

- [ ] a) defenses against specific threats.
- [ ] b) phagocytic activity for defense.
- [ ] c) complex, time-consuming defense mechanisms.
- [ ] d) immune surveillance.

10 The nonspecific defense that breaks down cells, attracts phagocytes, and stimulates inflammation is

- [ ] a) the inflammatory response.
- [ ] b) the action of interferons.
- [ ] c) the complement system.
- [ ] d) immune surveillance.

11 The protein(s) that interfere with the replication of viruses is (are)

- [ ] a) complement proteins.
- [ ] b) heparin.
- [ ] c) pyrogens.
- [ ] d) interferons.

12 Circulating proteins that reset the thermostat in the hypothalamus, causing a rise in body temperature, are called

- [ ] a) pyrogens.
- [ ] b) interferons.
- [ ] c) lysosomes.
- [ ] d) complement proteins.

13 The "first line of cellular defense" against pathogenic invasion is

- [ ] a) phagocytes.
- [ ] b) mucus.
- [ ] c) hair.
- [ ] d) interferon.

Short answer

We usually associate a fever with illness or disease. How can a fever be beneficial?

14 _____

Matching

Match each lettered term with the most closely related description.

a. opsonization

b. helper T cells

c. antibody

d. Class II MHC

e. costimulation

f. IgM

g. Class I MHC

h. IgG

i. passive immunity

j. anaphylaxis

k. CD4 markers

l. acquired immunity

m. B lymphocytes

1 Two parallel pairs of polypeptide chains

2 Found on helper T cells

3 Active and passive

4 Transfer of antibodies

5 Attacked by HIV

6 Enhances phagocytosis

7 MHC proteins present in the plasma membranes of all nucleated cells

8 Differentiate into memory and plasma cells

9 MHC proteins present in the plasma membranes of all APCs and lymphocytes

10 Antibodies used to determine blood type

11 Secondary binding process required for T cell activation

12 Accounts for 80 percent of all immunoglobulins

13 Circulating allergen stimulates mast cells throughout body

1 _____
2 _____
3 _____
4 _____
5 _____
6 _____
7 _____
8 _____
9 _____
10 _____
11 _____
12 _____
13 _____

Match each lettered term with the most closely related description.

a. cytotoxic T cells

b. viruses

c. B cells

d. antibodies

e. helper T cells

f. macrophages

g. natural killer (NK) cells

h. suppressor T cells

i. memory T cells and B cells

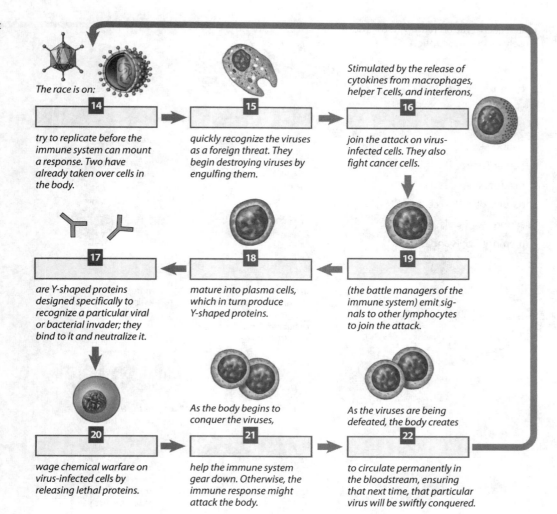

The race is on:

14 try to replicate before the immune system can mount a response. Two have already taken over cells in the body.

15 quickly recognize the viruses as a foreign threat. They begin destroying viruses by engulfing them.

Stimulated by the release of cytokines from macrophages, helper T cells, and interferons,

16 join the attack on virus-infected cells. They also fight cancer cells.

17 are Y-shaped proteins designed specifically to recognize a particular viral or bacterial invader; they bind to it and neutralize it.

18 mature into plasma cells, which in turn produce Y-shaped proteins.

19 (the battle managers of the immune system) emit signals to other lymphocytes to join the attack.

20 wage chemical warfare on virus-infected cells by releasing lethal proteins.

As the body begins to conquer the viruses,

21 help the immune system gear down. Otherwise, the immune response might attack the body.

As the viruses are being defeated, the body creates

22 to circulate permanently in the bloodstream, ensuring that next time, that particular virus will be swiftly conquered.

Matching

Match each lettered term with the most closely related description.

a. opsonization

b. helper T cells

c. antibody

d. Class II MHC

e. costimulation

f. IgM

g. Class I MHC

h. IgG

i. passive immunity

j. anaphylaxis

k. CD4 markers

l. acquired immunity

m. B lymphocytes

1 Two parallel pairs of polypeptide chains

2 Found on helper T cells

3 Active and passive

4 Transfer of antibodies

5 Attacked by HIV

6 Enhances phagocytosis

7 MHC proteins present in the plasma membranes of all nucleated cells

8 Differentiate into memory and plasma cells

9 MHC proteins present in the plasma membranes of all APCs and lymphocytes

10 Antibodies used to determine blood type

11 Secondary binding process required for T cell activation

12 Accounts for 80 percent of all immunoglobulins

13 Circulating allergen stimulates mast cells throughout body

1 _____

2 _____

3 _____

4 _____

5 _____

6 _____

7 _____

8 _____

9 _____

10 _____

11 _____

12 _____

13 _____

Match each lettered term with the most closely related description.

a. cytotoxic T cells

b. viruses

c. B cells

d. antibodies

e. helper T cells

f. macrophages

g. natural killer (NK) cells

h. suppressor T cells

i. memory T cells and B cells

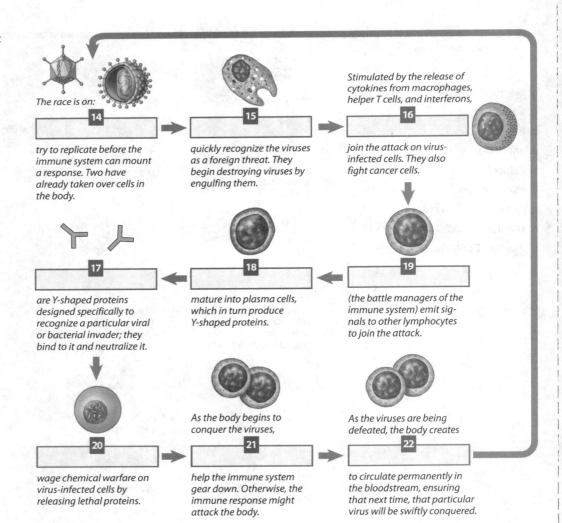

The race is on:

14 _____
try to replicate before the immune system can mount a response. Two have already taken over cells in the body.

15 _____
quickly recognize the viruses as a foreign threat. They begin destroying viruses by engulfing them.

Stimulated by the release of cytokines from macrophages, helper T cells, and interferons,
16 _____
join the attack on virus-infected cells. They also fight cancer cells.

17 _____
are Y-shaped proteins designed specifically to recognize a particular viral or bacterial invader; they bind to it and neutralize it.

18 _____
mature into plasma cells, which in turn produce Y-shaped proteins.

19 _____
(the battle managers of the immune system) emit signals to other lymphocytes to join the attack.

20 _____
wage chemical warfare on virus-infected cells by releasing lethal proteins.

As the body begins to conquer the viruses,
21 _____
help the immune system gear down. Otherwise, the immune response might attack the body.

As the viruses are being defeated, the body creates
22 _____
to circulate permanently in the bloodstream, ensuring that next time, that particular virus will be swiftly conquered.

Chapter Review Questions

Labeling

Label the antibody molecule shown here.

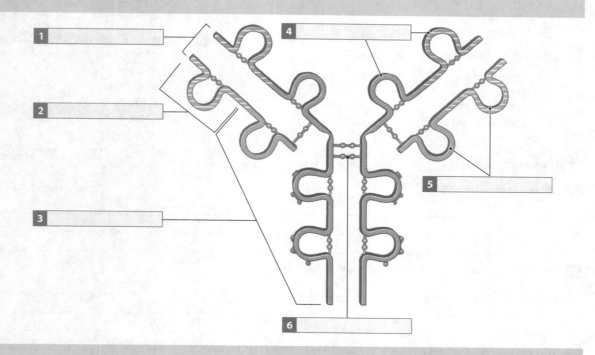

1 _____

2 _____

3 _____

4 _____

5 _____

6 _____

True/False

Indicate whether each statement is true or false.

7 One difference between lymphatic vessels and veins is that lymphatic vessels do not have valves.

8 Lymphopoiesis occurs exclusively in lymphoid tissue.

9 Efferent lymphatics arise from the hilum of a lymph node.

10 A decrease in circulating pyrogens results in an increase in body temperature.

11 Antibody molecules consist of four pairs of heavy chains and four pairs of light chains.

12 Under stimulation from cytokines, B cells can differentiate into plasma cells.

7 _____

8 _____

9 _____

10 _____

11 _____

12 _____

Multiple choice

Select the correct answer from the list provided.

13 Lymph from the left arm, the left half of the head, the left side of the body superior to the diaphragm, and the entire body inferior to the diaphragm is received by the
- a) thoracic duct.
- b) cisterna chyli.
- c) azygos vein.
- d) left lymphatic duct.

14 CD4 T cells respond to antigens presented by
- a) Class I MHC.
- b) Class II MHC.
- c) cytokines.
- d) plasma cells.

15 Interferons increase resistance of cells to
- a) fungal infections.
- b) bacterial infections.
- c) viral infections.
- d) cancer.

16 Which of the following immunoglobulins accounts for 80 percent of all antibodies?
- a) IgG
- b) IgE
- c) IgD
- d) IgM

17 The human immunodeficiency virus (HIV) infects which of the following cells?

☐ a) suppressor T cells

☐ b) memory T cells

☐ c) helper T cells

☐ d) cytotoxic T cells

18 Which of the following is *not* a phagocyte?

☐ a) neutrophil

☐ b) monocyte

☐ c) free macrophage

☐ d) natural killer cell

19 The adenoid is also known as the

☐ a) pharyngeal tonsil.

☐ b) palatine tonsil.

☐ c) lingual tonsil.

☐ d) Peyer's patch.

20 The gradual decrease in secretions and size of this organ with age is correlated with an increased susceptibility to disease.

☐ a) spleen

☐ b) thymus

☐ c) tonsils

☐ d) appendix

Short answer

21 What is graft rejection?

_____

_____

_____

22 How does a cytotoxic T cell (T_C cell) destroy its target cell?

_____

_____

_____

23 Why is it necessary for certain vaccinations, such as hepatitis B, to be administered as a series of injections over a period of months?

_____

_____

_____

Labeling

Label each of the respiratory system structures in the figure below.

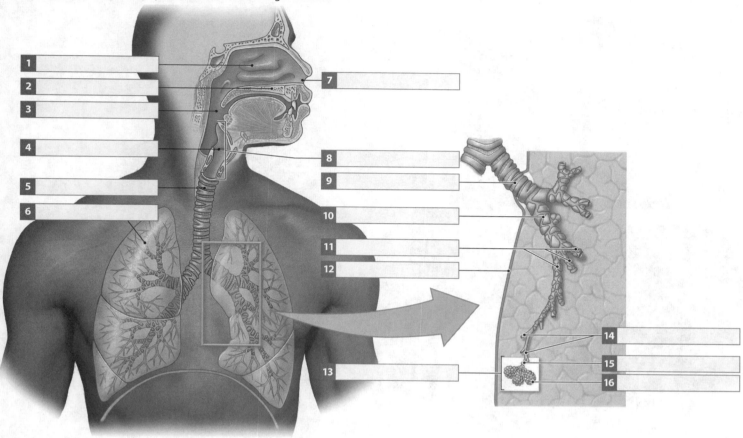

1.
2.
3.
4.
5.
6.
7.
8.
9.
10.
11.
12.
13.
14.
15.
16.

Matching

Match each lettered term with the most closely related description.

a. respiratory bronchiole

b. respiratory mucosa

c. phonation

d. bronchodilation

e. terminal bronchiole

f. laryngeal prominence

g. type I pneumocytes

h. type II pneumocytes

i. cystic fibrosis

j. trachea

k. pharynx

l. respiratory membrane

m. larynx

n. bronchoconstriction

17	Produce surfactant	17	____
18	Windpipe	18	____
19	Simple squamous epithelial cells	19	____
20	Sympathetic activation	20	____
21	Supplies a pulmonary lobule	21	____
22	Parasympathetic activation	22	____
23	Start of respiratory portion of respiratory tract	23	____
24	Gas exchange	24	____
25	Sound production at the larynx	25	____
26	Chamber shared by respiratory and digestive systems	26	____
27	Surrounds and protects the glottis	27	____
28	Lethal inherited respiratory disease	28	____
29	Lines the conducting portion of respiratory tract	29	____
30	Anterior surface of thyroid cartilage	30	____

Labeling

Label each of the respiratory system structures in the figure below.

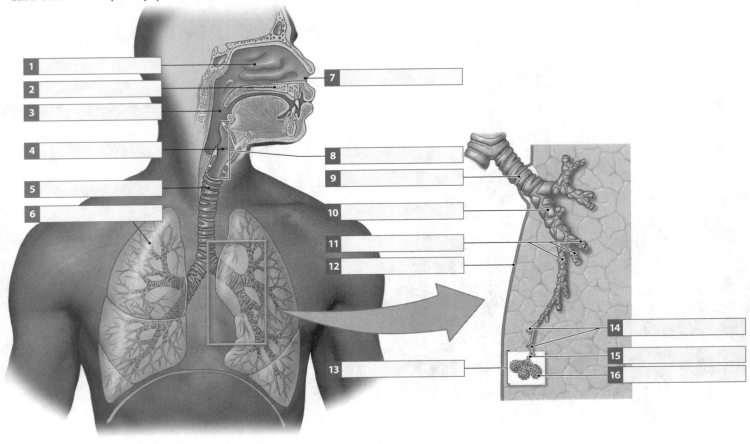

1 _____
2 _____
3 _____
4 _____
5 _____
6 _____
7 _____
8 _____
9 _____
10 _____
11 _____
12 _____
13 _____
14 _____
15 _____
16 _____

Matching

Match each lettered term with the most closely related description.

a. respiratory bronchiole
b. respiratory mucosa
c. phonation
d. bronchodilation
e. terminal bronchiole
f. laryngeal prominence
g. type I pneumocytes
h. type II pneumocytes
i. cystic fibrosis
j. trachea
k. pharynx
l. respiratory membrane
m. larynx
n. bronchoconstriction

17	Produce surfactant
18	Windpipe
19	Simple squamous epithelial cells
20	Sympathetic activation
21	Supplies a pulmonary lobule
22	Parasympathetic activation
23	Start of respiratory portion of respiratory tract
24	Gas exchange
25	Sound production at the larynx
26	Chamber shared by respiratory and digestive systems
27	Surrounds and protects the glottis
28	Lethal inherited respiratory disease
29	Lines the conducting portion of respiratory tract
30	Anterior surface of thyroid cartilage

17 _____
18 _____
19 _____
20 _____
21 _____
22 _____
23 _____
24 _____
25 _____
26 _____
27 _____
28 _____
29 _____
30 _____

Matching

Match each lettered term with the most closely related description.

a. apnea	**1** Single gas in a mixture	**1** _____
b. hemoglobin releases more O_2	**2** A cause of tissue death	**2** _____
c. lowers vital capacity	**3** Inverse pressure/volume relationship	**3** _____
d. external intercostals	**4** Expandability of lungs	**4** _____
e. iron ion	**5** CO_2 transport	**5** _____
f. Boyle's law	**6** Elastic tissue deterioration	**6** _____
g. compliance	**7** Act to elevate ribs	**7** _____
h. bicarbonate ion	**8** Heme unit	**8** _____
i. anoxia	**9** Blood pH decreases	**9** _____
j. atelectasis	**10** Promotes passive or active exhalation	**10** _____
k. hypocapnia	**11** Stimulate DRG and promotes inhalation	**11** _____
l. pneumotaxic centers	**12** Hyperventilation	**12** _____
m. apneustic centers	**13** Collapsed lung	**13** _____
n. partial pressure	**14** Period of suspended respiration	**14** _____

Short answer

Identify and describe the various pulmonary volumes and capacities indicated in the spirogram below.

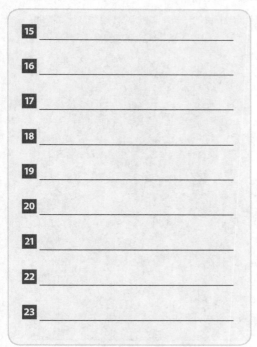

15 _____

16 _____

17 _____

18 _____

19 _____

20 _____

21 _____

22 _____

23 _____

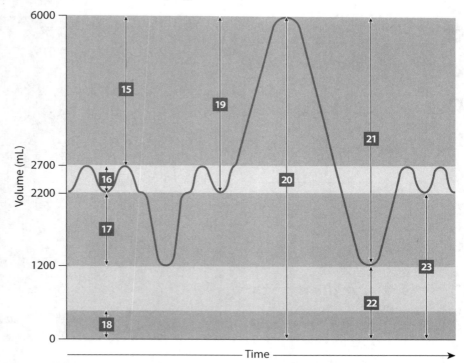

Section integration

Compare and contrast external respiration, pulmonary ventilation, and internal respiration.

24 _____

_____

Matching

Match each lettered term with the most closely related description.

a. apnea
b. hemoglobin releases more O_2
c. lowers vital capacity
d. external intercostals
e. iron ion
f. Boyle's law
g. compliance
h. bicarbonate ion
i. anoxia
j. atelectasis
k. hypocapnia
l. pneumotaxic centers
m. apneustic centers
n. partial pressure

1 Single gas in a mixture
2 A cause of tissue death
3 Inverse pressure/volume relationship
4 Expandability of lungs
5 CO_2 transport
6 Elastic tissue deterioration
7 Act to elevate ribs
8 Heme unit
9 Blood pH decreases
10 Promotes passive or active exhalation
11 Stimulate DRG and promotes inhalation
12 Hyperventilation
13 Collapsed lung
14 Period of suspended respiration

1 _____
2 _____
3 _____
4 _____
5 _____
6 _____
7 _____
8 _____
9 _____
10 _____
11 _____
12 _____
13 _____
14 _____

Short answer

Identify and describe the various pulmonary volumes and capacities indicated in the spirogram below.

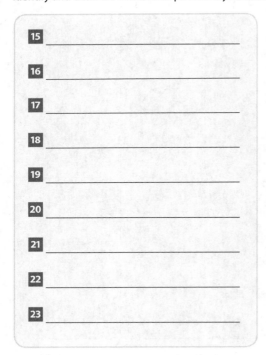

15 _____
16 _____
17 _____
18 _____
19 _____
20 _____
21 _____
22 _____
23 _____

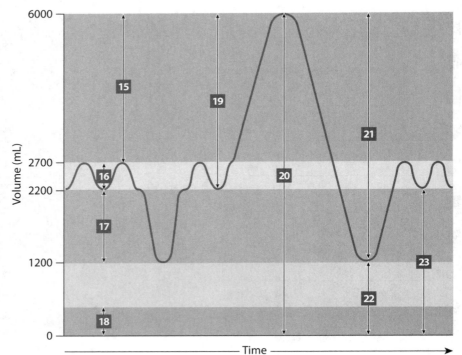

Section integration

Compare and contrast external respiration, pulmonary ventilation, and internal respiration.

24 _____

Chapter Review Questions

Labeling

Provide the values, in millimeters of mercury (mm Hg), on this illustration of the partial pressures of oxygen and carbon dioxide during external respiration in the pulmonary circuit and internal respiration in the systemic circuit.

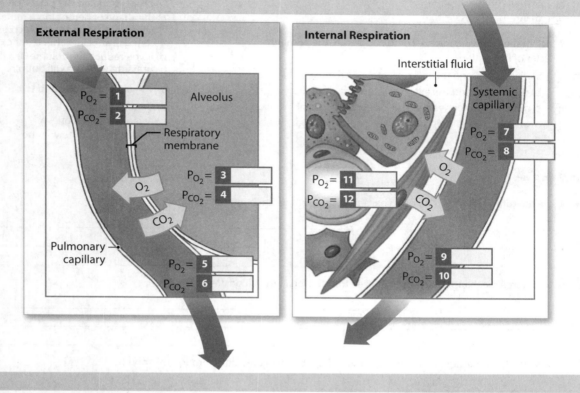

External Respiration

$P_{O_2} = $ [1]   Alveolus
$P_{CO_2} = $ [2]

— Respiratory membrane

$P_{O_2} = $ [3]
$P_{CO_2} = $ [4]

O_2

CO_2

Pulmonary capillary

$P_{O_2} = $ [5]
$P_{CO_2} = $ [6]

Internal Respiration

Interstitial fluid

Systemic capillary

$P_{O_2} = $ [7]
$P_{CO_2} = $ [8]

O_2

$P_{O_2} = $ [11]
$P_{CO_2} = $ [12]

CO_2

$P_{O_2} = $ [9]
$P_{CO_2} = $ [10]

Matching

Match each lettered term with the most closely related description.

a. respiratory rate
b. heme unit of Hb molecule
c. left lung
d. increasing pH
e. pulmonary ventilation
f. vital capacity
g. total lung capacity
h. right lung
i. globular unit of Hb molecule
j. respiratory minute volume
k. resistance
l. alveolar ventilation

13	Airflow to and from lungs	13	_____
14	Volume of air reaching alveoli each minute	14	_____
15	Has two lobes	15	_____
16	Binds CO_2	16	_____
17	Volume of air moved into and out of lungs each minute	17	_____
18	Binds O_2	18	_____
19	Number of breaths each minute	19	_____
20	Hb molecule releases less O_2	20	_____
21	Force required to inflate/deflate lungs	21	_____
22	Maximum amount of air moved into and out of lungs in one respiratory cycle	22	_____
23	Has three lobes	23	_____
24	Vital capacity plus residual volume	24	_____

Multiple choice

Select the correct answer from the list provided.

25 Surfactant
- [ ] a) protects the outer surface of the lungs.
- [ ] b) phagocytizes small particles.
- [ ] c) replaces mucus in the alveoli.
- [ ] d) helps prevent the alveoli from collapsing.

26 One of the responses to an abnormally low P_{CO_2} would be
- [ ] a) decreased respiratory rate.
- [ ] b) increased respiratory rate.
- [ ] c) hypercapnea.
- [ ] d) chronic obstructive pulmonary disease.

27 The narrow opening in the larynx for inhaled air is called the
- [ ] a) epiglottis.
- [ ] b) rima glottidis.
- [ ] c) pharynx.
- [ ] d) internal nares.

28 Which of the following muscle combinations are the primary muscles of inspiration?
- [ ] a) diaphragm and the internal intercostal muscles
- [ ] b) diaphragm and the external intercostal muscles
- [ ] c) abdominal muscles and the internal intercostal muscles
- [ ] d) abdominal muscles and the external intercostal muscles

29 Boyle's law states that
- [ ] a) all the partial pressures in a gas mixture added together equals the total pressure exerted by the gas mixture.
- [ ] b) the amount of a particular gas in solution is directly proportional to the partial pressure of that gas.
- [ ] c) the shape of hemoblogin molecules changes as the number of bound O_2 molecules increases, and these changes affect its affinity for oxygen.
- [ ] d) if you reduce the volume of a flexible container by half, the pressure within it will double.

30 $V_E = f \times V_T$ is the formula used to calculate
- [ ] a) Dalton's law.
- [ ] b) alveolar ventilation.
- [ ] c) respiratory minute volume.
- [ ] d) vital capacity.

Short answer

31 Name the three regions of the pharynx, and identify where each region is located.

_____

_____

_____

32 By what three mechanisms is carbon dioxide transported in the bloodstream?

_____

_____

33 Why is breathing through the nasal cavity more desirable than breathing through the mouth?

_____

_____

_____

Labeling

Label the structures of the digestive tract in the accompanying figure.

1 _____

2 _____

3 _____

4 _____

5 _____

6 _____

7 _____

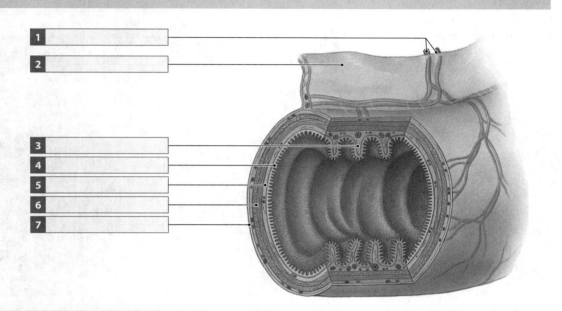

Matching

Match each lettered term with the most closely related description.

a. lamina propria

b. peristalsis

c. pacesetter cells

d. esophagus

e. muscularis mucosa

f. segmentation

g. circular folds

h. sphincter

i. myenteric plexus

j. visceral smooth muscle cells

k. plasticity

l. liver

m. multi-unit smooth muscle cells

n. bolus

8 Digestive tube between the pharynx and stomach

9 Moves circular folds and villi

10 Areolar tissue layer containing blood vessels, nerve endings, and lymphatics

11 Permanent transverse folds in the digestive tract lining

12 Waves of muscular contractions that propel materials along digestive tract

13 Stimulate rhythmic cycles of activity along digestive tract

14 Nerve network within the muscularis externa

15 Have direct contact with motor neurons

16 Digestive system accessory organ

17 Rhythmic muscular contractions that mix materials in digestive tract

18 Form of food entering the digestive tract

19 Lack direct contact with motor neurons

20 Ability of smooth muscle cells to function over varied lengths

21 Ring of muscle tissue

8 _____

9 _____

10 _____

11 _____

12 _____

13 _____

14 _____

15 _____

16 _____

17 _____

18 _____

19 _____

20 _____

21 _____

Section integration

How would a decrease in smooth muscle tone affect the digestive processes and possibly cause constipation (infrequent bowel movement)?

22 _____

_____

_____

Labeling

Label the structures of the digestive tract in the accompanying figure.

1 _____
2 _____

3 _____
4 _____
5 _____
6 _____
7 _____

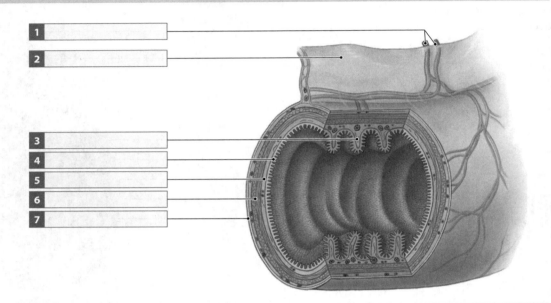

Matching

Match each lettered term with the most closely related description.

a. lamina propria
b. peristalsis
c. pacesetter cells
d. esophagus
e. muscularis mucosa
f. segmentation
g. circular folds
h. sphincter
i. myenteric plexus
j. visceral smooth muscle cells
k. plasticity
l. liver
m. multi-unit smooth muscle cells
n. bolus

8 Digestive tube between the pharynx and stomach
9 Moves circular folds and villi
10 Areolar tissue layer containing blood vessels, nerve endings, and lymphatics
11 Permanent transverse folds in the digestive tract lining
12 Waves of muscular contractions that propel materials along digestive tract
13 Stimulate rhythmic cycles of activity along digestive tract
14 Nerve network within the muscularis externa
15 Have direct contact with motor neurons
16 Digestive system accessory organ
17 Rhythmic muscular contractions that mix materials in digestive tract
18 Form of food entering the digestive tract
19 Lack direct contact with motor neurons
20 Ability of smooth muscle cells to function over varied lengths
21 Ring of muscle tissue

8 _____
9 _____
10 _____
11 _____
12 _____
13 _____
14 _____
15 _____
16 _____
17 _____
18 _____
19 _____
20 _____
21 _____

Section integration

How would a decrease in smooth muscle tone affect the digestive processes and possibly cause constipation (infrequent bowel movement)?

22 _____
_____
_____

Labeling

Label the structures of a typical tooth in the accompanying figure.

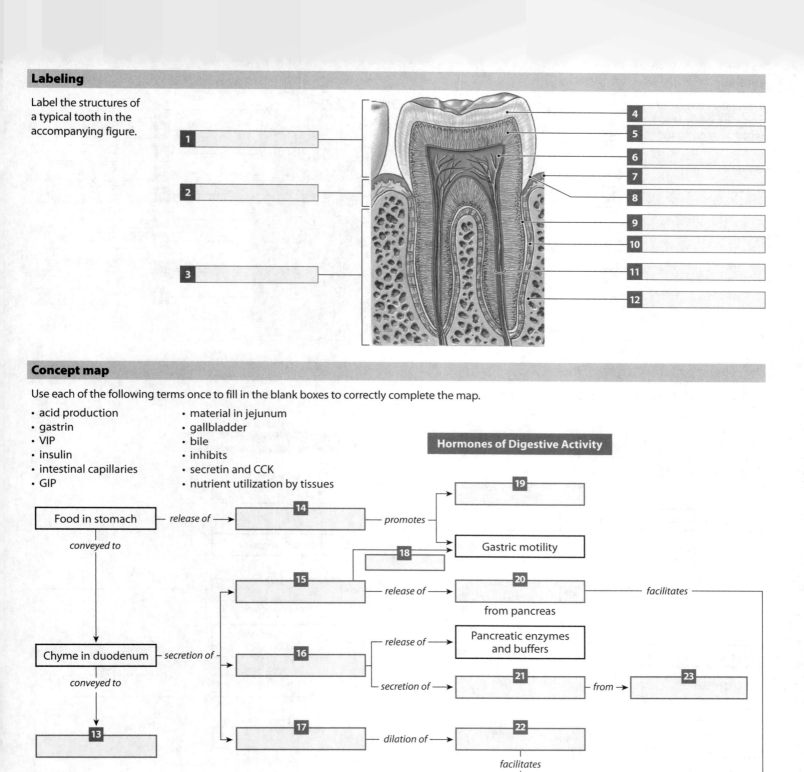

1	
2	
3	

4	
5	
6	
7	
8	
9	
10	
11	
12	

Concept map

Use each of the following terms once to fill in the blank boxes to correctly complete the map.

- acid production
- gastrin
- VIP
- insulin
- intestinal capillaries
- GIP
- material in jejunum
- gallbladder
- bile
- inhibits
- secretin and CCK
- nutrient utilization by tissues

Hormones of Digestive Activity

Food in stomach —*release of*→ [14] —*promotes*→ [19]

Food in stomach —*conveyed to*→ Chyme in duodenum

[18] → Gastric motility

[14] —*promotes*→ Gastric motility

Chyme in duodenum —*secretion of*→ [15] —*release of*→ [20] *from pancreas* —*facilitates*→ [24]

[15] → [18]

Chyme in duodenum —*conveyed to*→ [13]

[16] —*release of*→ Pancreatic enzymes and buffers

[16] —*secretion of*→ [21] —*from*→ [23]

[17] —*dilation of*→ [22] —*facilitates*→ Nutrient absorption

Short answer

Briefly describe the similarities and differences between parietal cells and chief cells in the stomach wall.

25 _____

_____

Labeling

Label the structures of a typical tooth in the accompanying figure.

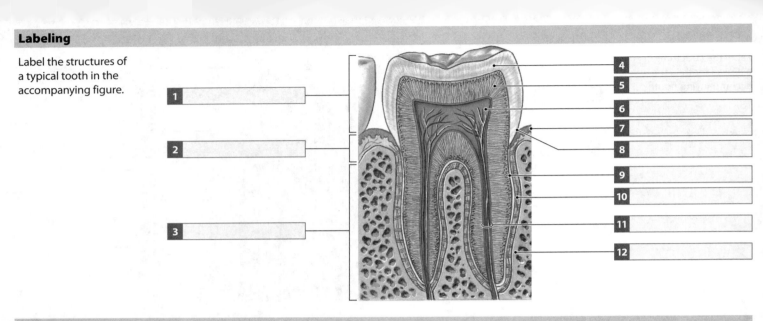

1. _____
2. _____
3. _____

4. _____
5. _____
6. _____
7. _____
8. _____
9. _____
10. _____
11. _____
12. _____

Concept map

Use each of the following terms once to fill in the blank boxes to correctly complete the map.

- acid production
- gastrin
- VIP
- insulin
- intestinal capillaries
- GIP
- material in jejunum
- gallbladder
- bile
- inhibits
- secretin and CCK
- nutrient utilization by tissues

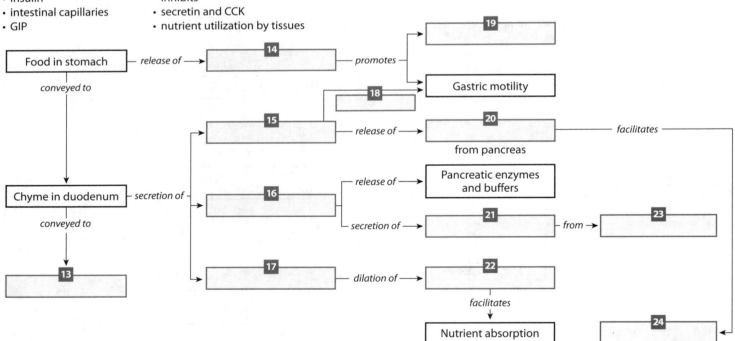

Hormones of Digestive Activity

Food in stomach — *release of* → 14 — *promotes* → 19

conveyed to

18 → Gastric motility

15 — *release of* → 20 from pancreas — *facilitates* →

Chyme in duodenum — *secretion of* → 16 — *release of* → Pancreatic enzymes and buffers

conveyed to

16 — *secretion of* → 21 — *from* → 23

13

17 — *dilation of* → 22

facilitates

↓

Nutrient absorption

24

Short answer

Briefly describe the similarities and differences between parietal cells and chief cells in the stomach wall.

25. _____

_____

Labeling

Label the structures of a liver lobule in the accompanying figure.

1 _____

2 _____

3 _____

4 _____

5 _____

9 _____

6 _____

7 _____

8 _____

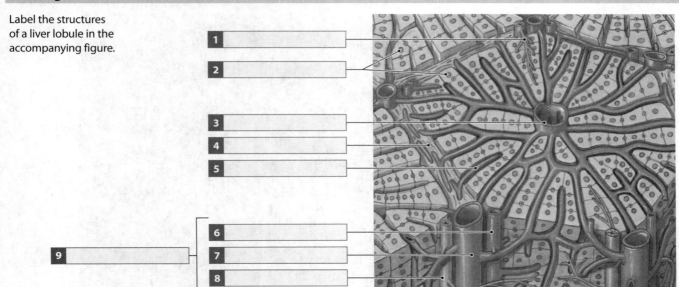

Matching

Match each lettered term with the most closely related description.

a. lysozyme

b. emulsification

c. gallstones

d. Kupffer cells

e. pancreatic lipase

f. liver

g. starch

h. pancreas

i. submandibular glands

j. hepatocytes

k. gallbladder

l. mumps

m. common bile duct

n. peptic ulcer

10 Pancreatic alpha-amylase substrate

11 Retroperitoneal organ

12 Drains liver and gallbladder

13 Bile-secreting cells

14 Viral infection of salivary glands

15 Digestive epithelial damage by acids

16 Process of breaking lipid droplets apart

17 Pancreatic enzyme that breaks down complex lipids

18 Organ that secretes bile continuously

19 Antibacterial enzyme

20 Greatest producer of saliva

21 Phagocytize and store iron

22 Stores bile

23 Cholecystitis

10 _____

11 _____

12 _____

13 _____

14 _____

15 _____

16 _____

17 _____

18 _____

19 _____

20 _____

21 _____

22 _____

23 _____

Short answer

Describe the beneficial roles of saliva.

24 _____

Section integration

Predict the consequences of a blockage of the duodenal ampulla by a tumor.

25 _____

Labeling

Label the structures of a liver lobule in the accompanying figure.

1 _____

2 _____

3 _____

4 _____

5 _____

6 _____

7 _____

8 _____

9 _____

Matching

Match each lettered term with the most closely related description.

a. lysozyme

b. emulsification

c. gallstones

d. Kupffer cells

e. pancreatic lipase

f. liver

g. starch

h. pancreas

i. submandibular glands

j. hepatocytes

k. gallbladder

l. mumps

m. common bile duct

n. peptic ulcer

10 Pancreatic alpha-amylase substrate

11 Retroperitoneal organ

12 Drains liver and gallbladder

13 Bile-secreting cells

14 Viral infection of salivary glands

15 Digestive epithelial damage by acids

16 Process of breaking lipid droplets apart

17 Pancreatic enzyme that breaks down complex lipids

18 Organ that secretes bile continuously

19 Antibacterial enzyme

20 Greatest producer of saliva

21 Phagocytize and store iron

22 Stores bile

23 Cholecystitis

10 _____

11 _____

12 _____

13 _____

14 _____

15 _____

16 _____

17 _____

18 _____

19 _____

20 _____

21 _____

22 _____

23 _____

Short answer

Describe the beneficial roles of saliva.

24 _____

Section integration

Predict the consequences of a blockage of the duodenal ampulla by a tumor.

25 _____

Chapter Review Questions

Labeling

Label the figure shown here.

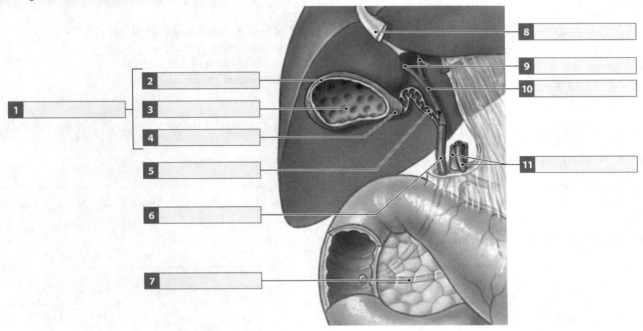

1	
2	
3	
4	
5	
6	
7	
8	
9	
10	
11	

True/False

Indicate whether each statement is true or false.

12 Kupffer cells are phagocytic cells within liver sinusoids.

13 The gallbladder produces almost as much bile on a daily basis as the liver.

14 Pancreatic islets produce the exocrine secretions for digestion.

15 Most saliva originates in the submandibular glands.

16 The correct order of small intestine segments is: duodenum, ileum, and jejunum.

17 Haustra are a series of pouches along the length of the colon.

12 _____

13 _____

14 _____

15 _____

16 _____

17 _____

Multiple choice

Select the correct answer from the list provided.

18 The release of pancreatic secretions and bile into the duodenum is caused by
- ☐ a) cholecystokinin.
- ☐ b) gastric inhibitory peptide.
- ☐ c) gastrin.
- ☐ d) vasoactive intestinal peptide.

19 Which of the following is *not* a major function of the large intestine?
- ☐ a) reabsorbing water and compacting the intestinal contents into feces
- ☐ b) producing enzymes that assist pancreatic juice
- ☐ c) absorbing vitamins produced by bacterial action
- ☐ d) storing fecal material prior to defecation

20 Fingerlike projections into the lumen of the small intestine are called

- ☐ a) microvilli.
- ☐ b) villi.
- ☐ c) circular folds.
- ☐ d) rugae.

21 A mesentery that forms a pouch between the body wall and the anterior surface of the small intestine is the

- ☐ a) greater omentum.
- ☐ b) lesser omentum.
- ☐ c) mesocolon.
- ☐ d) mesentery proper.

22 Pepsin is formed by a reaction between

- ☐ a) gastric lipase and acid.
- ☐ b) pepsinogen and intrinsic factors.
- ☐ c) bile and pancreatic juice.
- ☐ d) pepsinogen and acid.

23 Which of the following structures is *not* a component of a portal area?

- ☐ a) branch of the hepatic portal vein
- ☐ b) branch of the hepatic vein
- ☐ c) branch of the hepatic artery proper
- ☐ d) branch of a bile duct

Short answer

24 Name the four different types of teeth. What is the number of deciduous teeth and permanent teeth?

_____

_____

_____

25 Identify the three phases of gastric secretion, and provide a brief description of each phase.

_____

_____

_____

26 Describe the hepatic portal system.

_____

_____

_____

Matching

Match each lettered term with the appropriate numbered blank in the cellular metabolism figure to the right.

a. glucose
b. electron transport system
c. O_2
d. fatty acids
e. proteins
f. citric acid cycle
g. ATP
h. CO_2
i. H_2O
j. coenzymes
k. two-carbon chains

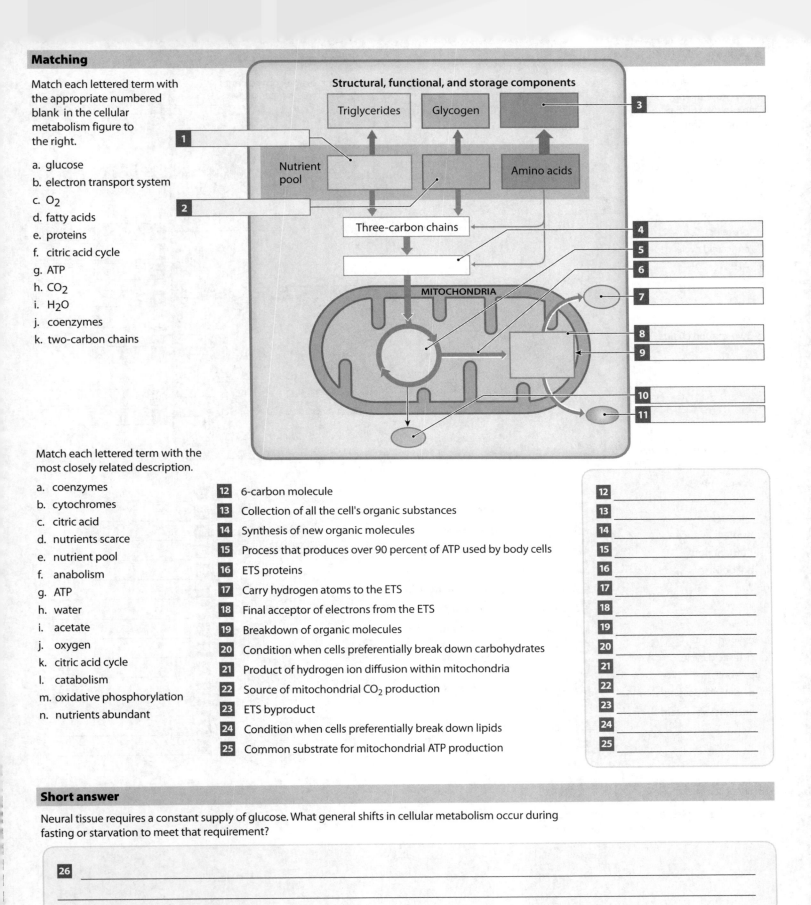

Structural, functional, and storage components

Triglycerides   Glycogen

3

1

Nutrient pool

2

Amino acids

Three-carbon chains

4

5

6

MITOCHONDRIA

7

8

9

10

11

Match each lettered term with the most closely related description.

a. coenzymes
b. cytochromes
c. citric acid
d. nutrients scarce
e. nutrient pool
f. anabolism
g. ATP
h. water
i. acetate
j. oxygen
k. citric acid cycle
l. catabolism
m. oxidative phosphorylation
n. nutrients abundant

12 6-carbon molecule

13 Collection of all the cell's organic substances

14 Synthesis of new organic molecules

15 Process that produces over 90 percent of ATP used by body cells

16 ETS proteins

17 Carry hydrogen atoms to the ETS

18 Final acceptor of electrons from the ETS

19 Breakdown of organic molecules

20 Condition when cells preferentially break down carbohydrates

21 Product of hydrogen ion diffusion within mitochondria

22 Source of mitochondrial CO_2 production

23 ETS byproduct

24 Condition when cells preferentially break down lipids

25 Common substrate for mitochondrial ATP production

12 _____
13 _____
14 _____
15 _____
16 _____
17 _____
18 _____
19 _____
20 _____
21 _____
22 _____
23 _____
24 _____
25 _____

Short answer

Neural tissue requires a constant supply of glucose. What general shifts in cellular metabolism occur during fasting or starvation to meet that requirement?

26 _____

_____

Matching

Match each lettered term with the appropriate numbered blank in the cellular metabolism figure to the right.

a. glucose
b. electron transport system
c. O_2
d. fatty acids
e. proteins
f. citric acid cycle
g. ATP
h. CO_2
i. H_2O
j. coenzymes
k. two-carbon chains

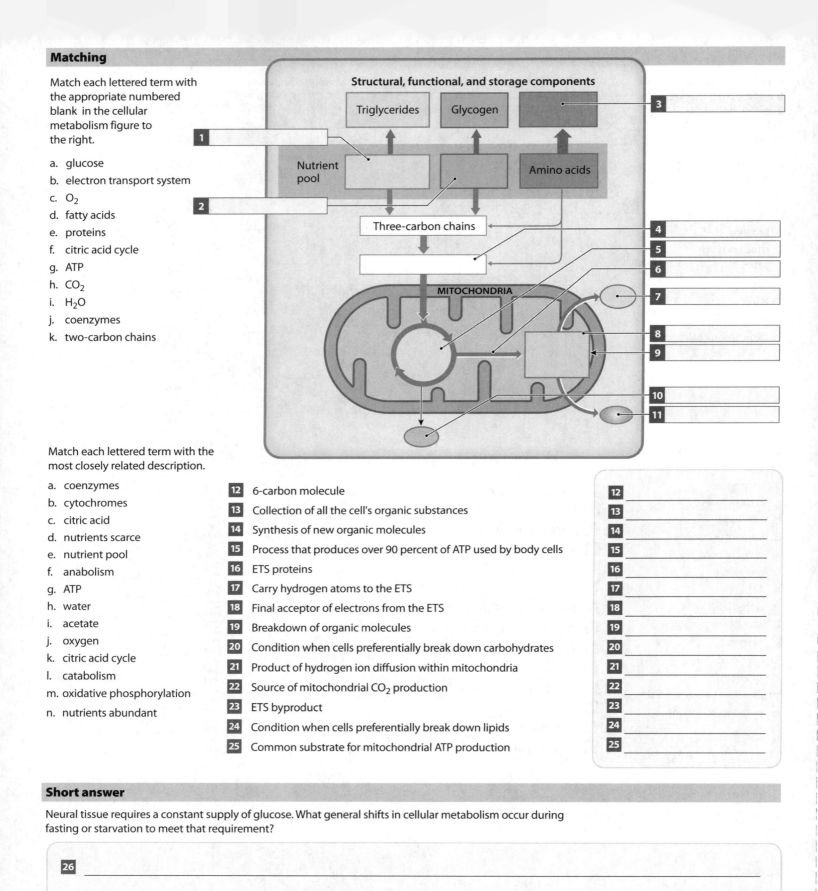

Structural, functional, and storage components

Triglycerides   Glycogen   ☐ 3

1 ☐

Nutrient pool   ☐   ☐   Amino acids

2 ☐

Three-carbon chains   ← 4

☐   5

☐   6

MITOCHONDRIA   ☐ 7

8

9

10

11

Match each lettered term with the most closely related description.

a. coenzymes
b. cytochromes
c. citric acid
d. nutrients scarce
e. nutrient pool
f. anabolism
g. ATP
h. water
i. acetate
j. oxygen
k. citric acid cycle
l. catabolism
m. oxidative phosphorylation
n. nutrients abundant

12	6-carbon molecule	12 _____
13	Collection of all the cell's organic substances	13 _____
14	Synthesis of new organic molecules	14 _____
15	Process that produces over 90 percent of ATP used by body cells	15 _____
16	ETS proteins	16 _____
17	Carry hydrogen atoms to the ETS	17 _____
18	Final acceptor of electrons from the ETS	18 _____
19	Breakdown of organic molecules	19 _____
20	Condition when cells preferentially break down carbohydrates	20 _____
21	Product of hydrogen ion diffusion within mitochondria	21 _____
22	Source of mitochondrial CO_2 production	22 _____
23	ETS byproduct	23 _____
24	Condition when cells preferentially break down lipids	24 _____
25	Common substrate for mitochondrial ATP production	25 _____

Short answer

Neural tissue requires a constant supply of glucose. What general shifts in cellular metabolism occur during fasting or starvation to meet that requirement?

26 _____

_____

Matching

Match each lettered term with the most closely related description.

a.	lipogenesis	**1**	Absorptive state hormone	**1**	_____
b.	anorexia	**2**	Glycogen reserves	**2**	_____
c.	lipolysis	**3**	Water-soluble vitamins	**3**	_____
d.	A, D, E, K	**4**	Fat catabolism	**4**	_____
e.	absorptive state	**5**	Lipid synthesis	**5**	_____
f.	deamination	**6**	Amino acid catabolism	**6**	_____
g.	ketone bodies	**7**	Fat-soluble vitamins	**7**	_____
h.	calorie	**8**	Lipid transport	**8**	_____
i.	uric acid	**9**	Removal of amino group	**9**	_____
j.	B complex and C	**10**	Lipid breakdown	**10**	_____
k.	urea formation	**11**	Gout	**11**	_____
l.	lipoproteins	**12**	Unit of energy	**12**	_____
m.	insulin	**13**	Period following a meal	**13**	_____
n.	skeletal muscle	**14**	Lack or loss of appetite	**14**	_____

Multiple choice

Select the correct answer from the list provided.

15 Intestinal absorption of nutrients occurs in the
- a) duodenum.
- b) ileocecum.
- c) ileum.
- d) jejunum.

16 When blood glucose concentrations are elevated, the glucose molecules are
- a) catabolized for energy.
- b) used to build protein.
- c) used for tissue repair.
- d) all of these

17 Most of the lipids absorbed by the digestive tract are immediately transferred to the
- a) liver.
- b) red blood cells.
- c) hepatocytes for storage.
- d) venous circulation by the thoracic duct.

18 Hypervitaminosis involving water-soluble vitamins is relatively uncommon because
- a) the excess amount is stored in adipose tissue.
- b) the excess amount is readily excreted in the urine.
- c) the excess amount is stored in the bones.
- d) excess amounts are readily absorbed by skeletal muscle tissue.

Short answer

19 What is the difference between an essential amino acid and a non-essential amino acid?

19 _____

20 Describe four reasons why protein catabolism is an impractical source of quick energy.

20 _____

21 What is the primary difference between the absorptive and postabsorptive states?

21 _____

22 Why is the liver the focal point for metabolic regulation and control?

22 _____

Section integration

Claudia suffers from anorexia nervosa. One afternoon she is rushed to the emergency room because of cardiac arrhythmias. Her breath smells fruity, and her blood and urine samples contain high levels of ketone bodies. Why does her breath have a fruity smell, and what would be the pH of her blood and urine?

23 _____

Matching

Match each lettered term with the most closely related description.

a. lipogenesis	1	Absorptive state hormone	1	_____
b. anorexia	2	Glycogen reserves	2	_____
c. lipolysis	3	Water-soluble vitamins	3	_____
d. A, D, E, K	4	Fat catabolism	4	_____
e. absorptive state	5	Lipid synthesis	5	_____
f. deamination	6	Amino acid catabolism	6	_____
g. ketone bodies	7	Fat-soluble vitamins	7	_____
h. calorie	8	Lipid transport	8	_____
i. uric acid	9	Removal of amino group	9	_____
j. B complex and C	10	Lipid breakdown	10	_____
k. urea formation	11	Gout	11	_____
l. lipoproteins	12	Unit of energy	12	_____
m. insulin	13	Period following a meal	13	_____
n. skeletal muscle	14	Lack or loss of appetite	14	_____

Multiple choice

Select the correct answer from the list provided.

15 Intestinal absorption of nutrients occurs in the
- ☐ a) duodenum.
- ☐ b) ileocecum.
- ☐ c) ileum.
- ☐ d) jejunum.

16 When blood glucose concentrations are elevated, the glucose molecules are
- ☐ a) catabolized for energy.
- ☐ b) used to build protein.
- ☐ c) used for tissue repair.
- ☐ d) all of these

17 Most of the lipids absorbed by the digestive tract are immediately transferred to the
- ☐ a) liver.
- ☐ b) red blood cells.
- ☐ c) hepatocytes for storage.
- ☐ d) venous circulation by the thoracic duct.

18 Hypervitaminosis involving water-soluble vitamins is relatively uncommon because
- ☐ a) the excess amount is stored in adipose tissue.
- ☐ b) the excess amount is readily excreted in the urine.
- ☐ c) the excess amount is stored in the bones.
- ☐ d) excess amounts are readily absorbed by skeletal muscle tissue.

Short answer

19 What is the difference between an essential amino acid and a non-essential amino acid?

20 Describe four reasons why protein catabolism is an impractical source of quick energy.

21 What is the primary difference between the absorptive and postabsorptive states?

22 Why is the liver the focal point for metabolic regulation and control?

19 _____
_____

20 _____
_____

21 _____
_____

22 _____
_____

Section integration

Claudia suffers from anorexia nervosa. One afternoon she is rushed to the emergency room because of cardiac arrhythmias. Her breath smells fruity, and her blood and urine samples contain high levels of ketone bodies. Why does her breath have a fruity smell, and what would be the pH of her blood and urine?

23 _____

Matching

Match each lettered term with the most closely related description.

a. ghrelin

b. basal metabolic rate

c. 40 percent

d. leptin

e. insensible perspiration

f. inhibits feeding center

g. shivering thermogenesis

h. peripheral vasoconstriction

i. thermoregulation

j. sensible perspiration

k. neuropeptide Y

l. 60 percent

m. nonshivering thermogenesis

n. peripheral vasodilation

1 Sweat gland activity; heat loss

2 Adipose tissue hormone

3 Homeostatic control of body temperature

4 General role of satiety center

5 Release of hormones; increased metabolism

6 Percent of catabolic energy released as heat

7 Stimulation of vasomotor center

8 Appetite-regulating neurotransmitter

9 Resting energy expenditure

10 Stomach hormone

11 Percent of catabolic energy captured as ATP

12 Inhibition of vasomotor center

13 Lung and epithelial water loss

14 Result of increased skeletal muscle tone

1 _____

2 _____

3 _____

4 _____

5 _____

6 _____

7 _____

8 _____

9 _____

10 _____

11 _____

12 _____

13 _____

14 _____

Multiple choice

Select the correct answer from the list provided.

15 A person's BMR is influenced by their

☐ a) gender.
☐ b) body weight.
☐ c) age.
☐ d) all of these

16 The processes involved in heat transfer between the body and the environment are

☐ a) sensible, insensible, heat loss, and heat gain.
☐ b) radiation, conduction, convection, and evaporation.
☐ c) physiological responses and behavioral modifications.
☐ d) sensible, insensible, hormones, and heat conservation.

17 The primary mechanisms for increasing heat loss from the body include

☐ a) vasomotor and respiratory.
☐ b) sensible and insensible.
☐ c) physiological responses and behavioral modifications.
☐ d) acclimatization and vasomotor.

18 All of the following are responses to an increase in body temperature, except

☐ a) stimulation of the respiratory centers.
☐ b) stimulation of sweat glands.
☐ c) peripheral vasoconstriction.
☐ d) peripheral vasodilation.

19 If daily intake exceeds total energy demands, the excess energy is stored primarily as

☐ a) triglycerides in adipose tissue.
☐ b) lipoproteins in the liver.
☐ c) glycogen in the liver.
☐ d) glucose in the bloodstream.

20 All of the following factors suppress appetite, except

☐ a) low blood glucose levels.
☐ b) high blood glucose levels.
☐ c) leptin.
☐ d) stimulation of stretch receptors along the digestive tract.

Short answer

21 How can a person's energy expenditure at rest be estimated by monitoring their oxygen consumption?

22 Describe the responses generated by the heat-gain center.

23 Describe the heat-gain mechanisms involved in nonshivering thermogenesis.

21 _____

_____

22 _____

_____

_____

23 _____

_____

_____

_____

_____

Matching

Match each lettered term with the most closely related description.

a. ghrelin
b. basal metabolic rate
c. 40 percent
d. leptin
e. insensible perspiration
f. inhibits feeding center
g. shivering thermogenesis
h. peripheral vasoconstriction
i. thermoregulation
j. sensible perspiration
k. neuropeptide Y
l. 60 percent
m. nonshivering thermogenesis
n. peripheral vasodilation

1	Sweat gland activity; heat loss
2	Adipose tissue hormone
3	Homeostatic control of body temperature
4	General role of satiety center
5	Release of hormones; increased metabolism
6	Percent of catabolic energy released as heat
7	Stimulation of vasomotor center
8	Appetite-regulating neurotransmitter
9	Resting energy expenditure
10	Stomach hormone
11	Percent of catabolic energy captured as ATP
12	Inhibition of vasomotor center
13	Lung and epithelial water loss
14	Result of increased skeletal muscle tone

1 _____
2 _____
3 _____
4 _____
5 _____
6 _____
7 _____
8 _____
9 _____
10 _____
11 _____
12 _____
13 _____
14 _____

Multiple choice

Select the correct answer from the list provided.

15 A person's BMR is influenced by their
- a) gender.
- b) body weight.
- c) age.
- d) all of these

16 The processes involved in heat transfer between the body and the environment are
- a) sensible, insensible, heat loss, and heat gain.
- b) radiation, conduction, convection, and evaporation.
- c) physiological responses and behavioral modifications.
- d) sensible, insensible, hormones, and heat conservation.

17 The primary mechanisms for increasing heat loss from the body include
- a) vasomotor and respiratory.
- b) sensible and insensible.
- c) physiological responses and behavioral modifications.
- d) acclimatization and vasomotor.

18 All of the following are responses to an increase in body temperature, except
- a) stimulation of the respiratory centers.
- b) stimulation of sweat glands.
- c) peripheral vasoconstriction.
- d) peripheral vasodilation.

19 If daily intake exceeds total energy demands, the excess energy is stored primarily as
- a) triglycerides in adipose tissue.
- b) lipoproteins in the liver.
- c) glycogen in the liver.
- d) glucose in the bloodstream.

20 All of the following factors suppress appetite, except
- a) low blood glucose levels.
- b) high blood glucose levels.
- c) leptin.
- d) stimulation of stretch receptors along the digestive tract.

Short answer

21 How can a person's energy expenditure at rest be estimated by monitoring their oxygen consumption?

22 Describe the responses generated by the heat-gain center.

23 Describe the heat-gain mechanisms involved in nonshivering thermogenesis.

21 _____
_____

22 _____
_____

23 _____
_____
_____
_____
_____

Chapter Review Questions

True/False

Indicate whether each statement is true or false.

1 The chemical reactions within cells are collectively known as cellular anabolism.

2 The breakdown of glucose into two 3-carbon molecules is called glycolysis.

3 The energy yield for carbohydrates is 4.18 Cal/g.

4 Kwashiorkor occurs in adults when uric acid crystals form in body fluids, causing a specific type of arthritis.

5 Leptin is a hormone secreted by the gastric mucosa that stimulates appetite.

6 The average person has a BMR of 70 Cal/hour, or about 1680 Cal/day.

1	_____
2	_____
3	_____
4	_____
5	_____
6	_____

Multiple choice

Select the correct answer from the list provided.

7 Catabolism refers to

- ☐ a) the creation of a nutrient pool.
- ☐ b) the sum total of all chemical reactions in the body.
- ☐ c) the production of organic compounds.
- ☐ d) the breakdown of organic substrates.

8 The breakdown of glucose to pyruvate is

- ☐ a) anaerobic.
- ☐ b) aerobic.
- ☐ c) lipogenic.
- ☐ d) anabolic.

9 The process that produces 90 percent of the ATP used by our cells is

- ☐ a) glycolysis.
- ☐ b) the citric acid cycle.
- ☐ c) oxidative phosphorylation.
- ☐ d) thermoregulation.

10 Glucose synthesis from smaller carbon chains is known as

- ☐ a) glycolysis.
- ☐ b) gluconeogenesis.
- ☐ c) glycogenesis.
- ☐ d) glycogenolysis.

11 The net result of one turn of the citric acid cycle is

- ☐ a) 1 ATP.
- ☐ b) 2 ATP.
- ☐ c) 17 ATP.
- ☐ d) 34 ATP.

12 Which of the following is a protein deficiency disease?

- ☐ a) phenylketonuria
- ☐ b) kwashiorkor
- ☐ c) ketoacidosis
- ☐ d) gouty arthritis

13 The enzyme that breaks down complex carbohydrates into a mixture of disaccharides and trisaccharides in the mouth is

- ☐ a) pepsin.
- ☐ b) lingual lipase.
- ☐ c) sucrase.
- ☐ d) salivary amylase.

14 Which of the following is a water-soluble vitamin?

- ☐ a) vitamin A
- ☐ b) vitamin C
- ☐ c) vitamin D_3
- ☐ d) vitamin K

15 The hormone released by adipose tissues as they synthesize triglycerides is

- ☐ a) leptin.
- ☐ b) ghrelin.
- ☐ c) neuropeptide Y.
- ☐ d) insulin.

16 More than 50 percent of the heat you lose indoors is attributable to

- ☐ a) radiation.
- ☐ b) sensible perspiration.
- ☐ c) convection.
- ☐ d) conduction.

Short answer

17 Explain how catabolism and anabolism are "linked" by ATP.

_____

_____

18 What level of total cholesterol is considered elevated, and what are the health risks of elevated cholesterol?

_____

_____

19 What are the risks of too much vitamin intake, and which vitamins are most commonly involved?

_____

_____

20 Distinguish between a calorie, a kilocalorie, and a Calorie.

_____

_____

_____

Concept map

Use each of the following terms once to fill in the blank boxes to correctly complete the map.

- ureter
- proximal convoluted tubule
- glomerulus
- urinary bladder
- renal tubules
- papillary ducts
- major calyces
- renal medulla
- renal sinus
- nephrons

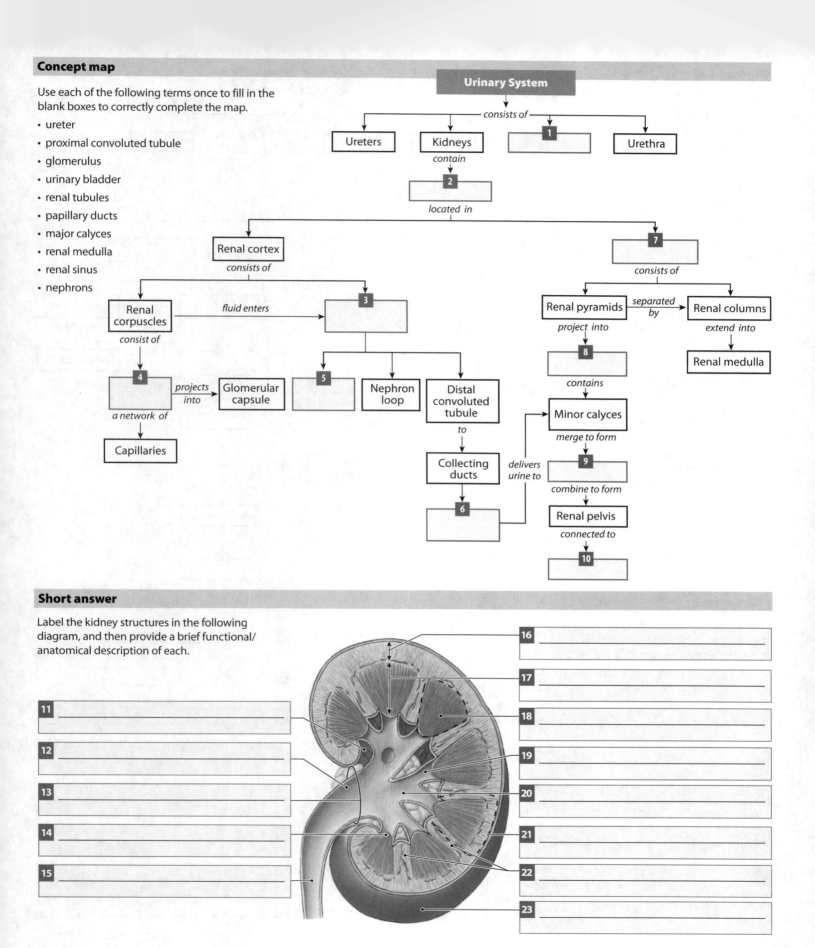

Urinary System

consists of

Ureters | Kidneys | **1** | Urethra

contain

2

located in

Renal cortex

consists of

7

consists of

Renal corpuscles — *fluid enters* → **3**

consist of

Renal pyramids — *separated by* → Renal columns

project into

extend into

4 — *projects into* → Glomerular capsule | **5** | Nephron loop | Distal convoluted tubule

8

Renal medulla

a network of

Capillaries

contains

to

Collecting ducts

Minor calyces

merge to form

9

combine to form

delivers urine to

6

Renal pelvis

connected to

10

Short answer

Label the kidney structures in the following diagram, and then provide a brief functional/anatomical description of each.

11 _____

12 _____

13 _____

14 _____

15 _____

16 _____

17 _____

18 _____

19 _____

20 _____

21 _____

22 _____

23 _____

175

Concept map

Use each of the following terms once to fill in the blank boxes to correctly complete the map.

- ureter
- proximal convoluted tubule
- glomerulus
- urinary bladder
- renal tubules
- papillary ducts
- major calyces
- renal medulla
- renal sinus
- nephrons

Urinary System

consists of

Ureters → Kidneys → [1] → Urethra

Kidneys *contain*

[2]

located in

Renal cortex

[7]

Renal cortex *consists of*

Renal corpuscles → *fluid enters* → [3]

[7] *consists of*

Renal pyramids → *separated by* → Renal columns

Renal pyramids *project into* → [8]

Renal columns *extend into* → Renal medulla

Renal corpuscles *consist of*

[4] → *projects into* → Glomerular capsule

[4] *a network of* → Capillaries

[3] → [5] / Nephron loop / Distal convoluted tubule

[8] *contains* → Minor calyces

Distal convoluted tubule *to* → Collecting ducts

Collecting ducts → *delivers urine to* → Minor calyces

Collecting ducts → [6]

Minor calyces *merge to form* → [9]

[9] *combine to form* → Renal pelvis

Renal pelvis *connected to* → [10]

Short answer

Label the kidney structures in the following diagram, and then provide a brief functional/anatomical description of each.

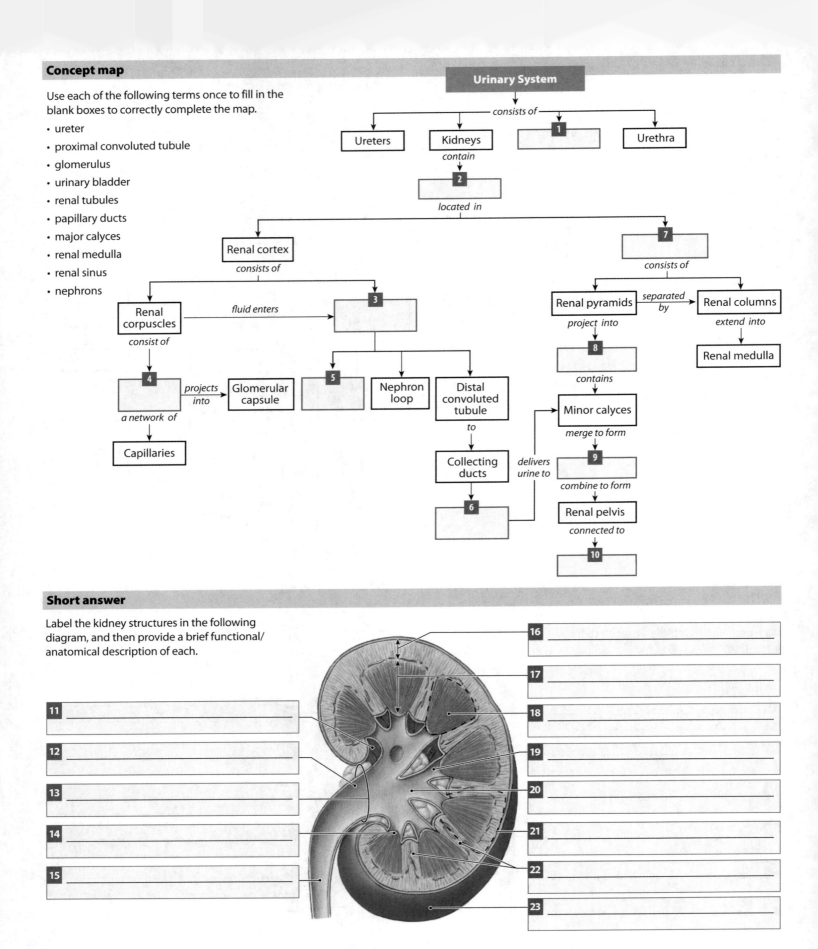

11 _____

12 _____

13 _____

14 _____

15 _____

16 _____

17 _____

18 _____

19 _____

20 _____

21 _____

22 _____

23 _____

Matching

Match each lettered term with the most closely related description.

a. aquaporins

b. ADH

c. aldosterone

d. PCT

e. secretion

f. renal corpuscle

g. nephron loop

h. filtrate

i. BCOP

j. podocytes

1	Site of plasma filtration	1 _____
2	Glomerular epithelium	2 _____
3	Protein-free solution	3 _____
4	Opposes filtration	4 _____
5	Countercurrent multiplication	5 _____
6	Water channels	6 _____
7	Primary method for eliminating drugs or toxins	7 _____
8	Stimulates ion pump—Na$^+$ reabsorbed	8 _____
9	Primary site of nutrient reabsorption in the nephron	9 _____
10	Regulates passive reabsorption of water from urine in the collecting system	10 _____

Short answer

Identify the structures of the representative nephron and collecting system in the following diagram, and describe the functions of each.

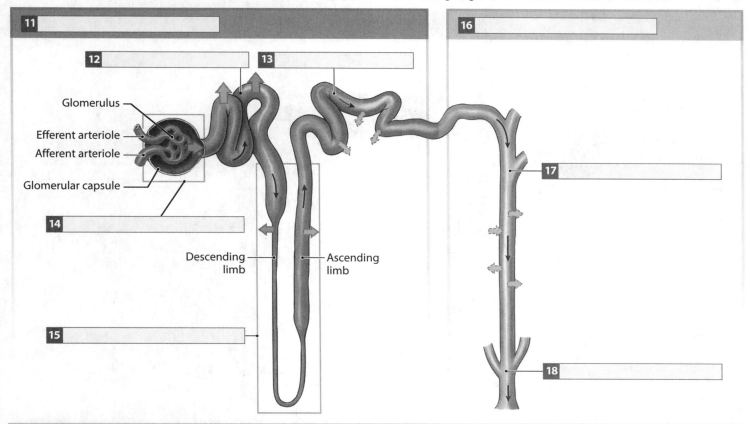

11 _____

16 _____

12 _____   13 _____

Glomerulus

Efferent arteriole

Afferent arteriole

Glomerular capsule

14 _____

17 _____

Descending limb   Ascending limb

15 _____

18 _____

Section integration

Marissa has had a urinalysis that detected large amounts of plasma proteins and white blood cells in her urine. What condition might be responsible, and what effects would it have on her urine output?

19 _____

_____

Matching

Match each lettered term with the most closely related description.

a. aquaporins

b. ADH

c. aldosterone

d. PCT

e. secretion

f. renal corpuscle

g. nephron loop

h. filtrate

i. BCOP

j. podocytes

1	Site of plasma filtration
2	Glomerular epithelium
3	Protein-free solution
4	Opposes filtration
5	Countercurrent multiplication
6	Water channels
7	Primary method for eliminating drugs or toxins
8	Stimulates ion pump—Na$^+$ reabsorbed
9	Primary site of nutrient reabsorption in the nephron
10	Regulates passive reabsorption of water from urine in the collecting system

1 _____

2 _____

3 _____

4 _____

5 _____

6 _____

7 _____

8 _____

9 _____

10 _____

Short answer

Identify the structures of the representative nephron and collecting system in the following diagram, and describe the functions of each.

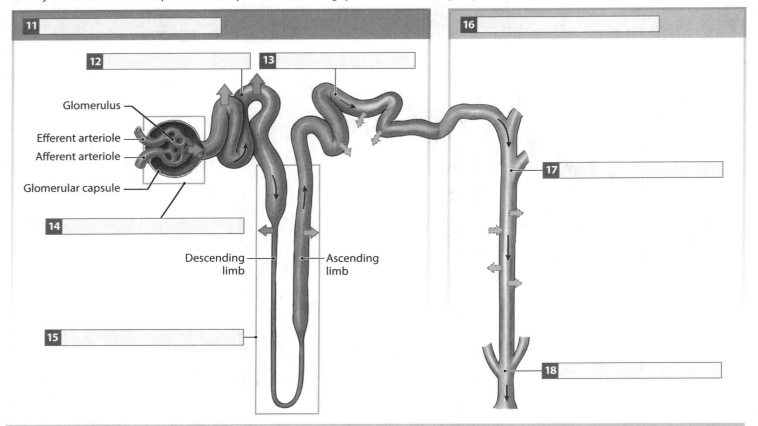

Section integration

Marissa has had a urinalysis that detected large amounts of plasma proteins and white blood cells in her urine. What condition might be responsible, and what effects would it have on her urine output?

19 _____

Labeling

Use the following descriptions to fill in the boxes in the micturition reflex diagram.

- sensation relayed to thalamus
- person relaxes external urethral sphincter
- afferent fibers carry information to sacral spinal cord
- sensation of bladder fullness delivered to cerebral cortex
- stretch receptors stimulated
- detrusor muscle contraction stimulated
- parasympathetic preganglionic fibers carry motor commands
- internal urethral sphincter relaxes

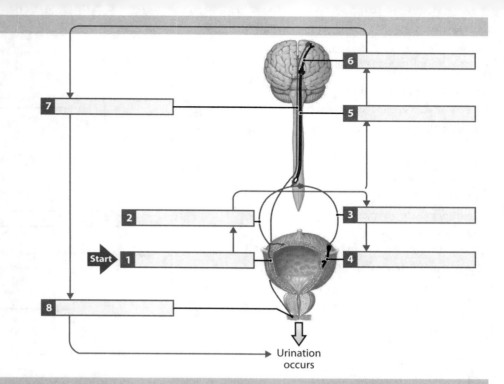

6 _____

7 _____

5 _____

2 _____

3 _____

Start 1 _____

4 _____

8 _____

Urination occurs

Matching

Match each lettered term with the most closely related description.

a. urethra
b. external urethral sphincter
c. detrusor
d. rugae
e. internal urethral sphincter
f. trigone
g. transitional epithelium
h. micturition
i. stratified squamous epithelium
j. external urethral orifice
k. middle umbilical ligament

9 The ring of smooth muscle in the neck of the urinary bladder
10 Triangular area within the urinary bladder
11 Relaxation of this muscle leads to urination
12 The external opening of the urethra
13 Folds lining the surface of the empty urinary bladder
14 Superior, supporting fibrous cord of the urinary bladder
15 Contraction of this smooth muscle compresses the urinary bladder
16 The type of epithelium that lines the ureters
17 Tube that transports urine to the exterior
18 Term for urination
19 Epithelium that lines the urethra

9 _____
10 _____
11 _____
12 _____
13 _____
14 _____
15 _____

16 _____
17 _____
18 _____
19 _____

Short answer

List four primary signs and symptoms of urinary disorders.

20 _____

Briefly describe the similarities and differences in the following pairs of terms.

21 cystitis/pyelonephritis
22 stress incontinence/overflow incontinence
23 polyuria/proteinuria

21 _____
22 _____
23 _____

Labeling

Use the following descriptions to fill in the boxes in the micturition reflex diagram.

- sensation relayed to thalamus
- person relaxes external urethral sphincter
- afferent fibers carry information to sacral spinal cord
- sensation of bladder fullness delivered to cerebral cortex
- stretch receptors stimulated
- detrusor muscle contraction stimulated
- parasympathetic preganglionic fibers carry motor commands
- internal urethral sphincter relaxes

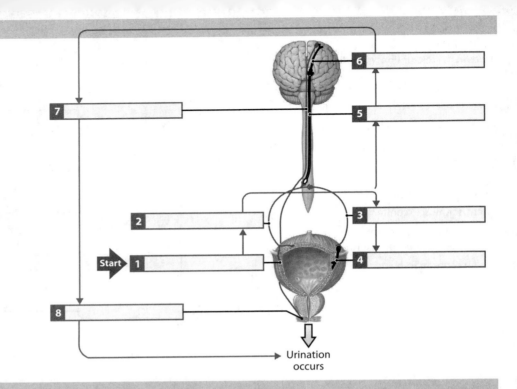

Urination occurs

Matching

Match each lettered term with the most closely related description.

a. urethra
b. external urethral sphincter
c. detrusor
d. rugae
e. internal urethral sphincter
f. trigone
g. transitional epithelium
h. micturition
i. stratified squamous epithelium
j. external urethral orifice
k. middle umbilical ligament

9 The ring of smooth muscle in the neck of the urinary bladder
10 Triangular area within the urinary bladder
11 Relaxation of this muscle leads to urination
12 The external opening of the urethra
13 Folds lining the surface of the empty urinary bladder
14 Superior, supporting fibrous cord of the urinary bladder
15 Contraction of this smooth muscle compresses the urinary bladder
16 The type of epithelium that lines the ureters
17 Tube that transports urine to the exterior
18 Term for urination
19 Epithelium that lines the urethra

9 _____
10 _____
11 _____
12 _____
13 _____
14 _____
15 _____

16 _____
17 _____
18 _____
19 _____

Short answer

List four primary signs and symptoms of urinary disorders.

20 _____

Briefly describe the similarities and differences in the following pairs of terms.

21 cystitis/pyelonephritis
22 stress incontinence/overflow incontinence
23 polyuria/proteinuria

21 _____
22 _____
23 _____

Chapter Review Questions

Labeling

Label the image of a renal corpuscle and associated structures shown here.

4		5	
1		6	
2		7	
3		8	

True/False

Indicate whether each statement is true or false.

9 The urinary tract includes the kidneys, ureters, urinary bladder, and urethra.

10 The left kidney lies slightly superior to the right kidney.

11 Most nephrons are cortical nephrons.

12 Tubular fluid is no longer modified beyond the DCT.

13 Contraction of the detrusor muscle moves urine along the ureters, toward the urinary bladder.

14 The process of urination is coordinated by the micturition reflex.

9 _____
10 _____
11 _____
12 _____
13 _____
14 _____

Multiple choice

Select the correct answer from the list provided.

15 The basic functional unit of the kidney is the
- ☐ a) filtration unit.
- ☐ b) nephron loop.
- ☐ c) glomerulus.
- ☐ d) nephron.

16 When ADH levels increase,
- ☐ a) the amount of water reabsorbed increases.
- ☐ b) the amount of water reabsorbed decreases.
- ☐ c) the DCT becomes impermeable to water.
- ☐ d) sodium ions are exchanged for potassium ions.

17 Which of the following conditions would cause an increase in the glomerular filtration rate?
- ☐ a) constriction of the afferent arteriole
- ☐ b) constriction of the efferent arteriole
- ☐ c) decrease in systemic blood pressure
- ☐ d) decrease in aldosterone and ADH production

18 Which of the following statements best describes the action of aldosterone at the DCT?
- ☐ a) Aldosterone stimulates actions that cause the secretion of drugs and toxins from the peritubular fluid.
- ☐ b) Sodium ions are reabsorbed in exchange for potassium ions by ion pumps stimulated by aldosterone.
- ☐ c) Aldosterone increases water secretion.
- ☐ d) Aldosterone causes glucose to be reabsorbed into the peritubular fluid.

19 Water reabsorption occurs primarily along the
- ☐ a) entire length of the nephron loop.
- ☐ b) ascending limb of the nephron loop and the DCT.
- ☐ c) PCT and descending limb of the nephron loop.
- ☐ d) DCT and collecting system.

20 In central regulation, decreased GFR is coordinated by the
- ☐ a) renal corpuscle.
- ☐ b) juxtamedullary complex.
- ☐ c) renal pelvis.
- ☐ d) cerebral cortex.

21 Urea is a byproduct of the breakdown of

- [ ] a) amino acids by the liver.
- [ ] b) creatine phosphate in skeletal muscle.
- [ ] c) the recycling of the nitrogenous bases in RNA molecules.
- [ ] d) glycogen to glucose.

22 Which of the following is *not* a response to angiotensin II?

- [ ] a) decreased ADH production
- [ ] b) increased stimulation of the thirst centers
- [ ] c) increased aldosterone secretion by the adrenal glands
- [ ] d) constriction of peripheral arteries and further constriction of the efferent arterioles

Short answer

23 Identify and describe the three distinct processes in urine production.

_____

_____

_____

24 Describe the primary process involved in glomerular filtration.

_____

_____

_____

25 What is countercurrent multiplication?

_____

_____

_____

Matching

Match each lettered term with the most closely related description.

a. kidneys
b. potassium
c. fluid compartments
d. fluid balance
e. hypertonic blood plasma
f. dehydration
g. aldosterone
h. plasma, interstitial fluid
i. osmoreceptors
j. fluid shift
k. hypokalemia
l. ADH
m. hyponatremia
n. sodium

1 Monitor blood osmotic concentration
2 Water gain = water loss
3 Major components of ECF
4 Dominant cation in ECF
5 Hormone that restricts water loss and stimulates thirst
6 Caused by overhydration
7 Dominant cation in ICF
8 ICF and ECF
9 Most important sites of sodium ion regulation
10 Water movement between ECF and ICF
11 Water moves from cells into ECF
12 Result of aldosteronism
13 Water losses greater than water gains
14 Regulates sodium ion absorption along distal convoluted tubule and collecting system

1 _____
2 _____
3 _____
4 _____
5 _____
6 _____
7 _____
8 _____
9 _____
10 _____
11 _____
12 _____
13 _____
14 _____

Multiple choice

Select the correct answer from the list provided.

15 Nearly two-thirds of the total body water content is
   a) extracellular fluid (ECF).
   b) intracellular fluid (ICF).
   c) tissue fluid.
   d) interstitial fluid.

16 Electrolyte balance involves balancing the rates of absorption across the digestive tract with rates of loss at the
   a) heart and lungs.
   b) stomach and liver.
   c) kidneys and sweat glands.
   d) pancreas and gallbladder.

17 If the ECF is hypertonic with respect to the ICF, water will move
   a) from the ECF into cells until osmotic equilibrium is restored.
   b) from cells into the ECF until osmotic equilibrium is restored.
   c) in both directions until osmotic equilibrium is restored.
   d) in response to the sodium–potassium exchange pump.

18 When pure water is consumed, the ECF
   a) becomes hypotonic with respect to the ICF.
   b) becomes hypertonic with respect to the ICF.
   c) becomes isotonic with respect to the ICF.
   d) electrolytes become more concentrated.

19 Physiological adjustments affecting fluid and electrolyte balance are mediated primarily by
   a) antidiuretic hormone.
   b) aldosterone.
   c) natriuretic peptides.
   d) all of the above

20 When water is lost but electrolytes are retained, the osmolarity of the ECF rises, and osmosis then moves water
   a) out of the ECF and into the ICF.
   b) back and forth between the ICF and ECF.
   c) out of the ICF and into the ECF.
   d) none of the above

Section integration

Malia, a nursing student, has been caring for burn patients. She notices that they consistently show elevated levels of potassium in their urine and wonders why. What would you tell her?

21 _____
_____

Matching

Match each lettered term with the most closely related description.

a. kidneys
b. potassium
c. fluid compartments
d. fluid balance
e. hypertonic blood plasma
f. dehydration
g. aldosterone
h. plasma, interstitial fluid
i. osmoreceptors
j. fluid shift
k. hypokalemia
l. ADH
m. hyponatremia
n. sodium

1	Monitor blood osmotic concentration
2	Water gain = water loss
3	Major components of ECF
4	Dominant cation in ECF
5	Hormone that restricts water loss and stimulates thirst
6	Caused by overhydration
7	Dominant cation in ICF
8	ICF and ECF
9	Most important sites of sodium ion regulation
10	Water movement between ECF and ICF
11	Water moves from cells into ECF
12	Result of aldosteronism
13	Water losses greater than water gains
14	Regulates sodium ion absorption along distal convoluted tubule and collecting system

1 _____
2 _____
3 _____
4 _____
5 _____
6 _____
7 _____
8 _____
9 _____
10 _____
11 _____
12 _____
13 _____
14 _____

Multiple choice

Select the correct answer from the list provided.

15 Nearly two-thirds of the total body water content is
  a) extracellular fluid (ECF).
  b) intracellular fluid (ICF).
  c) tissue fluid.
  d) interstitial fluid.

16 Electrolyte balance involves balancing the rates of absorption across the digestive tract with rates of loss at the
  a) heart and lungs.
  b) stomach and liver.
  c) kidneys and sweat glands.
  d) pancreas and gallbladder.

17 If the ECF is hypertonic with respect to the ICF, water will move
  a) from the ECF into cells until osmotic equilibrium is restored.
  b) from cells into the ECF until osmotic equilibrium is restored.
  c) in both directions until osmotic equilibrium is restored.
  d) in response to the sodium–potassium exchange pump.

18 When pure water is consumed, the ECF
  a) becomes hypotonic with respect to the ICF.
  b) becomes hypertonic with respect to the ICF.
  c) becomes isotonic with respect to the ICF.
  d) electrolytes become more concentrated.

19 Physiological adjustments affecting fluid and electrolyte balance are mediated primarily by
  a) antidiuretic hormone.
  b) aldosterone.
  c) natriuretic peptides.
  d) all of the above

20 When water is lost but electrolytes are retained, the osmolarity of the ECF rises, and osmosis then moves water
  a) out of the ECF and into the ICF.
  b) back and forth between the ICF and ECF.
  c) out of the ICF and into the ECF.
  d) none of the above

Section integration

Malia, a nursing student, has been caring for burn patients. She notices that they consistently show elevated levels of potassium in their urine and wonders why. What would you tell her?

21 _____

Labeling

Use the following terms to label the boxes in the two flowcharts. Terms may be used more than once.

- blood pH decrease
- blood pH increase
- increased P_{CO_2}
- decreased P_{CO_2}
- increased
- decreased
- alkalosis
- acidosis
- generated
- secreted

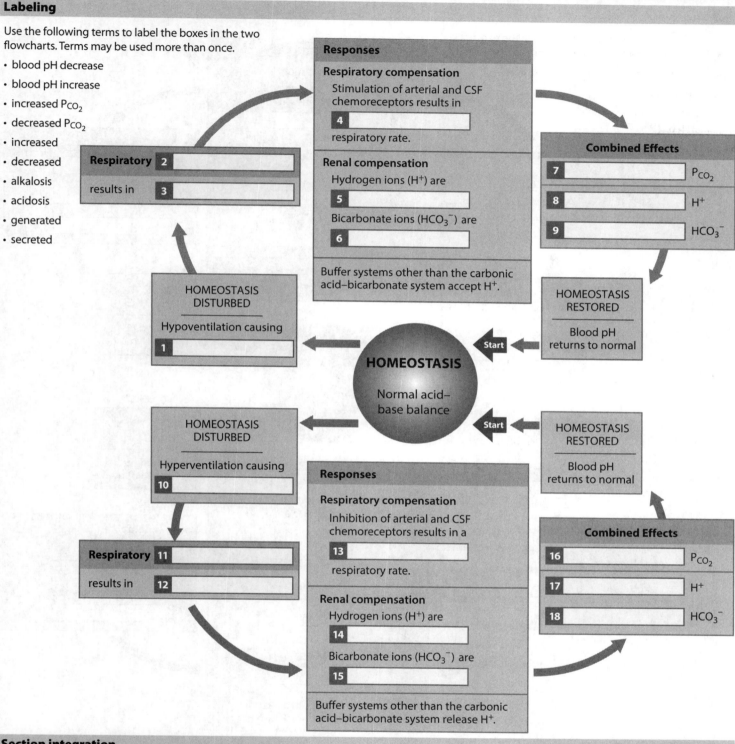

Responses

Respiratory compensation
Stimulation of arterial and CSF chemoreceptors results in [4] respiratory rate.

Renal compensation
Hydrogen ions (H^+) are [5]
Bicarbonate ions (HCO_3^-) are [6]

Buffer systems other than the carbonic acid–bicarbonate system accept H^+.

Combined Effects
[7] P_{CO_2}
[8] H^+
[9] HCO_3^-

Respiratory [2]
results in [3]

HOMEOSTASIS DISTURBED

Hypoventilation causing
[1]

HOMEOSTASIS RESTORED

Blood pH returns to normal

Start

HOMEOSTASIS
Normal acid–base balance

Start

HOMEOSTASIS RESTORED

Blood pH returns to normal

HOMEOSTASIS DISTURBED

Hyperventilation causing
[10]

Responses

Respiratory compensation
Inhibition of arterial and CSF chemoreceptors results in a [13] respiratory rate.

Renal compensation
Hydrogen ions (H^+) are [14]
Bicarbonate ions (HCO_3^-) are [15]

Buffer systems other than the carbonic acid–bicarbonate system release H^+.

Respiratory [11]
results in [12]

Combined Effects
[16] P_{CO_2}
[17] H^+
[18] HCO_3^-

Section integration

After falling into a deep lake and nearly drowning, a young boy is rescued. His rescuers assess his condition and find that his body fluids have high P_{CO_2} and lactate levels, and low P_{O_2} levels. Identify the underlying problem, and recommend the necessary treatment to restore homeostatic conditions.

[19] _____

Labeling

Use the following terms to label the boxes in the two flowcharts. Terms may be used more than once.

- blood pH decrease
- blood pH increase
- increased P_{CO_2}
- decreased P_{CO_2}
- increased
- decreased
- alkalosis
- acidosis
- generated
- secreted

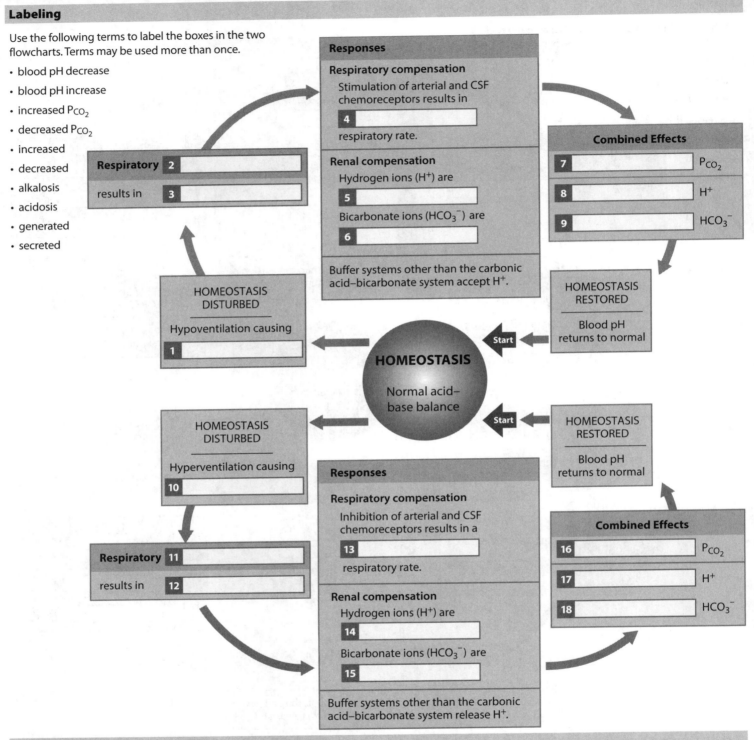

Section integration

After falling into a deep lake and nearly drowning, a young boy is rescued. His rescuers assess his condition and find that his body fluids have high P_{CO_2} and lactate levels, and low P_{O_2} levels. Identify the underlying problem, and recommend the necessary treatment to restore homeostatic conditions.

19 _____

Chapter Review Questions

True/False

Indicate whether each statement is true or false.

1. Metabolic acidosis develops when large numbers of hydrogen ions are removed from body fluids, resulting in an increase in pH.

2. Proteins are the most abundant solid components of body mass.

3. About half of daily water loss occurs through evaporation at the lungs.

4. Respiratory alkalosis can be treated by simply having the person breathe in and out of a paper bag.

5. Hypokalemia is caused by inadequate aldosterone secretion.

6. Iron is classified as a bulk mineral.

7. Carbonic acid is a volatile acid that forms through the interaction of water and carbon dioxide.

8. The pH of ECF normally ranges from 7.0 to 7.30.

9. The total body composition of adult males is 60 percent water and 40 percent solids, while for females, total body composition is 50 percent water and 50 percent solids.

10. About 98 percent of the potassium content of the human body is in the ICF, rather than the ECF.

1. _____

2. _____

3. _____

4. _____

5. _____

6. _____

7. _____

8. _____

9. _____

10. _____

Matching

Match each lettered term with the most closely related description.

a. buffer
b. acid
c. basic, or alkaline
d. pH
e. acidic
f. base
g. neutral
h. salt

11. The negative exponent of the hydrogen ion concentration in a solution

12. A substance that dissociates to release hydroxide ions or to remove hydrogen ions, increasing pH

13. A solution with a pH of 7; it contains equal numbers of hydrogen ions and hydroxide ions

14. A substance that tends to oppose changes in the pH of a solution by removing or replacing hydrogen ions

15. A solution with a pH above 7; hydroxide ions predominate

16. A substance that dissociates to release hydrogen ions, decreasing pH

17. An ionic compound consisting of a cation other than a hydrogen ion and an anion other than a hydroxide ion

18. A solution with a pH below 7; hydrogen ions predominate

11. _____

12. _____

13. _____

14. _____

15. _____

16. _____

17. _____

18. _____

Multiple choice

Select the correct answer from the list provided.

19 The most important factor affecting the pH of body tissues is the

- [ ] a) hydrochloric acid.
- [ ] b) ketone bodies.
- [ ] c) lactic acid.
- [ ] d) partial pressure of carbon dioxide.

20 Respiratory acidosis develops when the pH of blood is

- [ ] a) increased due to decreased P_{CO_2} level.
- [ ] b) decreased due to increased P_{CO_2} level.
- [ ] c) increased due to increased P_{CO_2} level.
- [ ] d) decreased due to decreased P_{CO_2} level.

21 Which of the following is the correct chemical equation of the reaction between water and carbon dioxide?

- [ ] a) $H_2CO_3 + H^+ \longrightarrow HCO_3^- + H_2O \longrightarrow CO_2$
- [ ] b) $H_2O + CO_2 \longrightarrow H_2CO_3 \longrightarrow H^+ + HCO_3^-$
- [ ] c) $H_2O + CO_2 \longrightarrow HCO_3^- \longrightarrow H_2CO_3 \longrightarrow H^+$
- [ ] d) $H_2O + CO_2 + H^+ \longrightarrow H_2CO_3 \longrightarrow HCO_3^-$

22 Most of the buffering capacity of proteins is provided by the

- [ ] a) R-groups of the component amino acids.
- [ ] b) peptide bonds between adjacent amino acids.
- [ ] c) amino and carboxyl groups of the component amino acids.
- [ ] d) central carbon group of most amino acids.

23 Which of the following is *not* an endocrine response to decreased blood volume and blood pressure?

- [ ] a) increased renin secretion and angiotensin II activation
- [ ] b) increased aldosterone release
- [ ] c) increased ADH release
- [ ] d) increased Na^+ in urine

24 The condition of below normal Na^+ concentration in the blood is called

- [ ] a) hyponatremia.
- [ ] b) hypernatremia.
- [ ] c) hypokalemia.
- [ ] d) hyperkalemia.

25 Which of the following minerals functions as a component of myoglobin, hemoglobin, and cytochromes?

- [ ] a) zinc
- [ ] b) copper
- [ ] c) iron
- [ ] d) cobalt

26 The primary site of ion loss is at the

- [ ] a) sweat glands.
- [ ] b) kidneys.
- [ ] c) intestines.
- [ ] d) lungs.

Short answer

27 Differentiate between fluid balance, mineral balance, and acid–base balance.

_____

_____

_____

28 What would happen if a dehydrated patient accidentally received an intravenous solution of hypertonic saline?

_____

_____

_____

Labeling

Label the structures of the male reproductive system in the accompanying diagram.

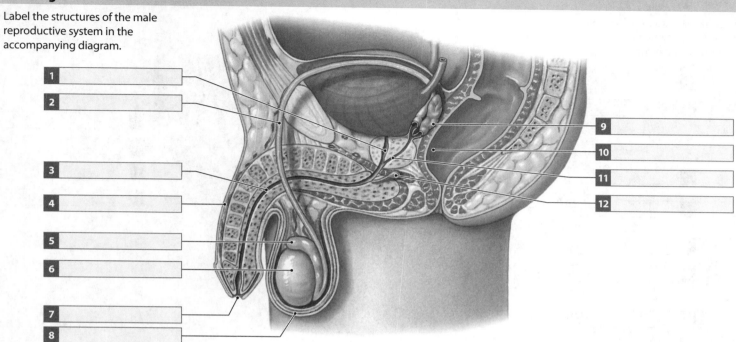

1 _____
2 _____
3 _____
4 _____
5 _____
6 _____
7 _____
8 _____

9 _____
10 _____
11 _____
12 _____

Matching

Match each lettered term with the most closely related description.

a. semen
b. epididymis
c. nurse cells
d. corpus spongiosum
e. luteinizing hormone (LH)
f. impotence
g. follicle-stimulating hormone (FSH)
h. spermatogonia
i. seminiferous tubules
j. dartos muscle
k. spermatogenesis
l. interstitial cells
m. spermiogenesis
n. penis and scrotum

13 Scrotal smooth muscle
14 Sperm stem cells
15 Sites of sperm production
16 Produce testosterone
17 Physical maturation of spermatids
18 Sperm production
19 External genitalia
20 Start of male reproductive tract
21 Maintain blood–testis barrier
22 Spermatozoa and seminal fluid
23 Inability to achieve or maintain an erection
24 Erectile tissue surrounding the urethra
25 Induces secretion of androgens
26 Hormone that targets nurse cells

13 _____
14 _____
15 _____
16 _____
17 _____
18 _____
19 _____
20 _____
21 _____
22 _____
23 _____
24 _____
25 _____
26 _____

Section integration

In males, the endocrine disorder hypogonadism is primarily due to the underproduction of testosterone or the lack of tissue sensitivity to testosterone, and results in sterility. What are five primary functions of testosterone in males?

27 _____

_____

Labeling

Label the structures of the male reproductive system in the accompanying diagram.

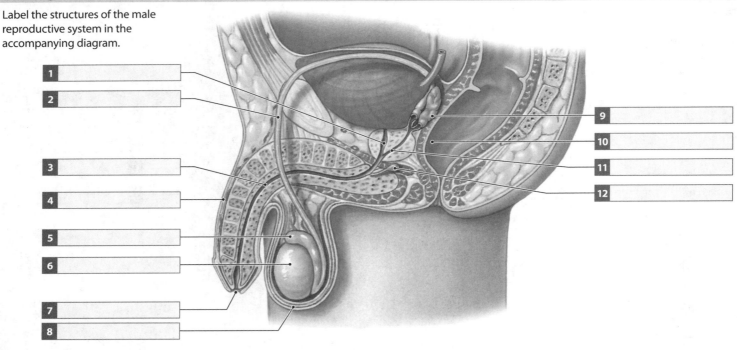

1 _____

2 _____

3 _____

4 _____

5 _____

6 _____

7 _____

8 _____

9 _____

10 _____

11 _____

12 _____

Matching

Match each lettered term with the most closely related description.

a. semen
b. epididymis
c. nurse cells
d. corpus spongiosum
e. luteinizing hormone (LH)
f. impotence
g. follicle-stimulating hormone (FSH)
h. spermatogonia
i. seminiferous tubules
j. dartos muscle
k. spermatogenesis
l. interstitial cells
m. spermiogenesis
n. penis and scrotum

13 Scrotal smooth muscle
14 Sperm stem cells
15 Sites of sperm production
16 Produce testosterone
17 Physical maturation of spermatids
18 Sperm production
19 External genitalia
20 Start of male reproductive tract
21 Maintain blood–testis barrier
22 Spermatozoa and seminal fluid
23 Inability to achieve or maintain an erection
24 Erectile tissue surrounding the urethra
25 Induces secretion of androgens
26 Hormone that targets nurse cells

13 _____
14 _____
15 _____
16 _____
17 _____
18 _____
19 _____
20 _____
21 _____
22 _____
23 _____
24 _____
25 _____
26 _____

Section integration

In males, the endocrine disorder hypogonadism is primarily due to the underproduction of testosterone or the lack of tissue sensitivity to testosterone, and results in sterility. What are five primary functions of testosterone in males?

27 _____

_____

Labeling

Label the structures of the female reproductive system in the accompanying diagram.

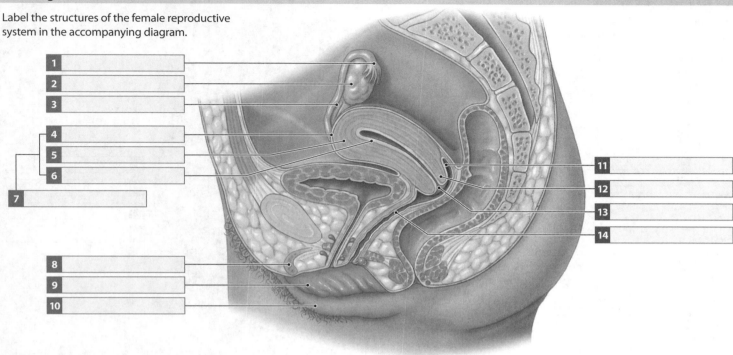

1	
2	
3	
4	
5	
6	
7	
8	
9	
10	
11	
12	
13	
14	

Matching

Match each lettered term with the most closely related description.

a. LH surge
b. rectouterine pouch
c. tubal ligation
d. menarche
e. ovaries
f. corpus luteum
g. vulva
h. cervix
i. broad ligament
j. oocytes
k. GnRH
l. vesicouterine pouch
m. lactation
n. uterine cycle

15 Immature female gametes
16 First menstrual cycle
17 Pocket anterior to the uterus
18 Encloses the ovaries, uterine tubes, and uterus
19 Pocket posterior to the uterus
20 Endocrine structure
21 Averages 28 days
22 Milk production
23 Oocyte and hormone production
24 Triggers ovulation
25 Inferior portion of the uterus
26 Female surgical sterilization
27 Stimulates FSH production and secretion
28 Contains female external genitalia

15 _____
16 _____
17 _____
18 _____
19 _____
20 _____
21 _____
22 _____
23 _____
24 _____
25 _____
26 _____
27 _____
28 _____

Section integration

In a condition known as endometriosis, endometrial cells migrate from the body of the uterus either into the uterine tubes or through the uterine tubes and into the peritoneal cavity, where they become established. Explain why periodic pain is a major symptom of endometriosis.

29 _____

_____

Labeling

Label the structures of the female reproductive system in the accompanying diagram.

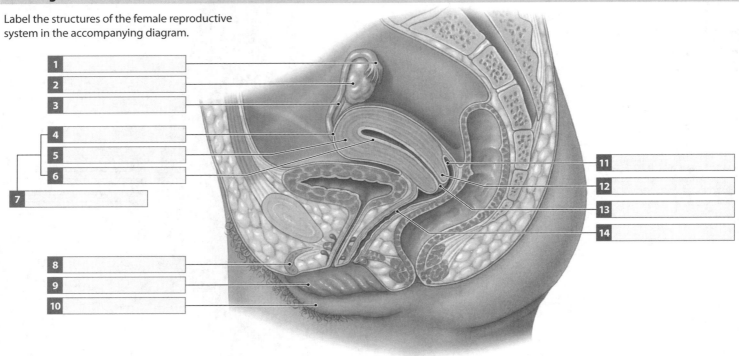

1	
2	
3	
4	
5	
6	
7	
8	
9	
10	
11	
12	
13	
14	

Matching

Match each lettered term with the most closely related description.

a. LH surge
b. rectouterine pouch
c. tubal ligation
d. menarche
e. ovaries
f. corpus luteum
g. vulva
h. cervix
i. broad ligament
j. oocytes
k. GnRH
l. vesicouterine pouch
m. lactation
n. uterine cycle

15	Immature female gametes	15	_____
16	First menstrual cycle	16	_____
17	Pocket anterior to the uterus	17	_____
18	Encloses the ovaries, uterine tubes, and uterus	18	_____
19	Pocket posterior to the uterus	19	_____
20	Endocrine structure	20	_____
21	Averages 28 days	21	_____
22	Milk production	22	_____
23	Oocyte and hormone production	23	_____
24	Triggers ovulation	24	_____
25	Inferior portion of the uterus	25	_____
26	Female surgical sterilization	26	_____
27	Stimulates FSH production and secretion	27	_____
28	Contains female external genitalia	28	_____

Section integration

In a condition known as endometriosis, endometrial cells migrate from the body of the uterus either into the uterine tubes or through the uterine tubes and into the peritoneal cavity, where they become established. Explain why periodic pain is a major symptom of endometriosis.

| 29 | _____ |
| | _____ |

Chapter Review Questions

Labeling

Label the male and female reproductive structures shown here.

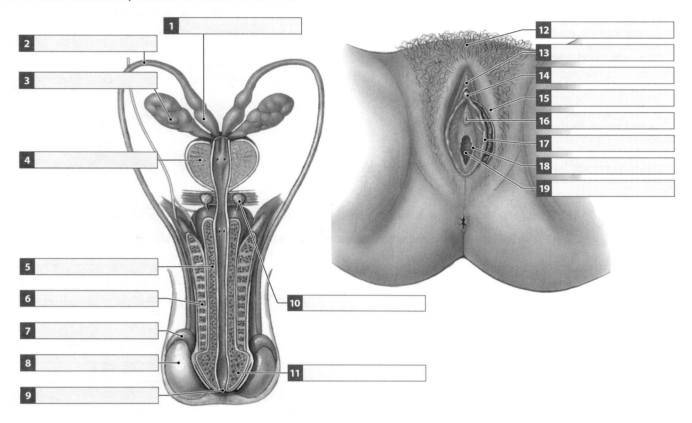

1	12
2	13
3	14
4	15
5	16
6	17
7	18
8	19
9	
10	
11	

True/False

Indicate whether each statement is true or false.

20 The prostate gland is the site of sperm maturation.

21 Secondary spermatocytes contain 23 chromosomes.

22 In the male, LH induces the secretion of testosterone and other androgens by the interstitial cells of the testes.

23 At the end of meiosis II in females, four functional oocytes are produced.

24 A massive surge of LH on or around day 14 of the menstrual cycle triggers ovulation and formation of the corpus luteum.

25 *Gardasil* is a vaccine that protects against the virus that causes about 75 percent of ovarian cancers.

20 _____

21 _____

22 _____

23 _____

24 _____

25 _____

Multiple choice

Select the correct answer from the list provided.

26 In females, meiosis II is not completed until
- ☐ a) birth.
- ☐ b) ovulation.
- ☐ c) fertilization.
- ☐ d) uterine implantation.

27 Progesterone secretion is performed by the
- ☐ a) primary follicle.
- ☐ b) secondary follicle.
- ☐ c) corpus luteum.
- ☐ d) corpus albicans.

28 Spermatogenesis begins with the division of spermatogonia in the

☐ a) epididymis.

☐ b) seminiferous tubules.

☐ c) ductus deferens.

☐ d) bulbourethral glands.

29 Erection of the penis is a result of

☐ a) parasympathetic neurons releasing nitric oxide at their axon terminals, causing the penile arteries to dilate, increasing blood flow to the penis.

☐ b) sympathetic neurons releasing nitric oxide at their axon terminals, causing the penile arteries to dilate, increasing blood flow to the penis.

☐ c) parasympathetic neurons releasing nitric oxide at their axon terminals, causing the penile veins to constrict, decreasing blood flow from the the penis.

☐ d) sympathetic neurons releasing nitric oxide at their axon terminals, causing the penile veins to constrict, decreasing blood flow from the penis.

30 Estrogens are produced by

☐ a) the zona pellucida and the corona radiata.

☐ b) primordial follicles and the zona pellucida.

☐ c) primary oocytes and cells of the corpus luteum.

☐ d) thecal cells and granulosa cells.

31 About 60 percent of the volume of semen is produced by the

☐ a) seminal glands.

☐ b) prostate gland.

☐ c) bulbourethral glands.

☐ d) ductus deferens.

Short answer

32 Explain how oral contraceptives that contain estrogen and progesterone, or only progesterone, prevent ovulation.

_____

_____

_____

33 What happens to the tertiary follicle after ovulation?

_____

_____

_____

34 Identify the sterilization procedures for men and women. How is sexual function affected as a result of each?

_____

_____

_____

Matching

Match each lettered term with the most closely related description.

a. hCG
b. conception
c. chorion
d. syncytial trophoblast
e. colostrum
f. amnion
g. amphimixis
h. morula
i. embryonic disc
j. neonate
k. gestation
l. inner cell mass
m. relaxin
n. blastocyst

1	Fertilization
2	Newborn infant
3	Pronuclei fuse
4	Period of prenatal development
5	Pregnancy test
6	Softens pubic symphysis
7	Mammary gland secretion
8	Mesoderm and ectoderm
9	Hollow ball of cells
10	Mesoderm and trophoblast
11	Forms the embryo
12	Cytoplasm with many nuclei
13	Solid ball of cells
14	Gastrulation product

1 _____
2 _____
3 _____
4 _____
5 _____
6 _____
7 _____
8 _____
9 _____
10 _____
11 _____
12 _____
13 _____
14 _____

Multiple choice

Select the correct answer from the list provided.

15 Fertilization typically occurs in the
- a) lower part of the uterine tube.
- b) upper part of the uterus.
- c) junction between the ampulla and isthmus of the uterine tube.
- d) cervix.

16 Fetal development begins at the start of the
- a) implantation process.
- b) second month after fertilization.
- c) ninth week after fertilization.
- d) sixth month after fertilization.

17 Organs and organ systems complete most of their development by the end of the
- a) first trimester.
- b) second trimester.
- c) third trimester.
- d) expulsion stage.

18 The four general processes that occur during the first trimester include
- a) blastomere, blastocyst, morula, and trophoblast.
- b) cleavage, implantation, placentation, and embryogenesis.
- c) placentation, dilation, expulsion, and organogenesis.
- d) yolk sac, amnion, allantois, and chorion.

19 The most dangerous period in prenatal or neonatal life is the
- a) first trimester.
- b) second trimester.
- c) third trimester.
- d) expulsion stage.

20 The systems that were relatively nonfunctional during the fetal period that must become functional at birth are the
- a) cardiovascular, muscular, and skeletal systems.
- b) integumentary, reproductive, and nervous systems.
- c) respiratory, digestive, and urinary systems.
- d) endocrine, nervous, and digestive systems.

Section integration

Tina gives birth to a baby with a congenital deformity of the stomach. Tina thinks her baby's condition resulted from a viral infection she had during her third trimester. Explain if the viral infection likely caused the baby's condition.

21 _____
_____

Matching

Match each lettered term with the most closely related description.

a. hCG	**1** Fertilization	**1** _____
b. conception	**2** Newborn infant	**2** _____
c. chorion	**3** Pronuclei fuse	**3** _____
d. syncytial trophoblast	**4** Period of prenatal development	**4** _____
e. colostrum	**5** Pregnancy test	**5** _____
f. amnion	**6** Softens pubic symphysis	**6** _____
g. amphimixis	**7** Mammary gland secretion	**7** _____
h. morula	**8** Mesoderm and ectoderm	**8** _____
i. embryonic disc	**9** Hollow ball of cells	**9** _____
j. neonate	**10** Mesoderm and trophoblast	**10** _____
k. gestation	**11** Forms the embryo	**11** _____
l. inner cell mass	**12** Cytoplasm with many nuclei	**12** _____
m. relaxin	**13** Solid ball of cells	**13** _____
n. blastocyst	**14** Gastrulation product	**14** _____

Multiple choice

Select the correct answer from the list provided.

15 Fertilization typically occurs in the
- ☐ a) lower part of the uterine tube.
- ☐ b) upper part of the uterus.
- ☐ c) junction between the ampulla and isthmus of the uterine tube.
- ☐ d) cervix.

16 Fetal development begins at the start of the
- ☐ a) implantation process.
- ☐ b) second month after fertilization.
- ☐ c) ninth week after fertilization.
- ☐ d) sixth month after fertilization.

17 Organs and organ systems complete most of their development by the end of the
- ☐ a) first trimester.
- ☐ b) second trimester.
- ☐ c) third trimester.
- ☐ d) expulsion stage.

18 The four general processes that occur during the first trimester include
- ☐ a) blastomere, blastocyst, morula, and trophoblast.
- ☐ b) cleavage, implantation, placentation, and embryogenesis.
- ☐ c) placentation, dilation, expulsion, and organogenesis.
- ☐ d) yolk sac, amnion, allantois, and chorion.

19 The most dangerous period in prenatal or neonatal life is the
- ☐ a) first trimester.
- ☐ b) second trimester.
- ☐ c) third trimester.
- ☐ d) expulsion stage.

20 The systems that were relatively nonfunctional during the fetal period that must become functional at birth are the
- ☐ a) cardiovascular, muscular, and skeletal systems.
- ☐ b) integumentary, reproductive, and nervous systems.
- ☐ c) respiratory, digestive, and urinary systems.
- ☐ d) endocrine, nervous, and digestive systems.

Section integration

Tina gives birth to a baby with a congenital deformity of the stomach. Tina thinks her baby's condition resulted from a viral infection she had during her third trimester. Explain if the viral infection likely caused the baby's condition.

21 _____

_____

Matching

Match each lettered term with the most closely related description.

a. genotype

b. heterozygous

c. locus

d. autosomes

e. simple inheritance

f. homozygous

g. alleles

h. polygenic inheritance

i. homologous

j. genetics

k. karyotype

l. phenotype

1 Visible characteristics

2 Alternate forms of a gene

3 Refers to the two members of a pair of chromosomes

4 Array of the entire set of chromosomes in a cell

5 An individual's chromosomes and genes

6 Gene's position on a chromosome

7 Two different alleles for the same gene

8 Study of the mechanisms of inheritance

9 Two identical alleles for the same gene

10 Interactions between alleles on several genes

11 Phenotype determined by a single pair of alleles

12 Chromosomes affecting somatic characteristics

1 _____

2 _____

3 _____

4 _____

5 _____

6 _____

7 _____

8 _____

9 _____

10 _____

11 _____

12 _____

Section integration

Using the templates below, draw Punnett squares to answer each question about the following genetic conditions.

13 Tongue-rolling is inherited as a strictly dominant trait. Using *T* for tongue-rolling and *t* for non-tongue-rolling, determine the possible genotypic and phenotypic ratios of offspring born to two heterozygous tongue-rolling parents. What is the probability they will have a child unable to roll his/her tongue?

14 Cystic fibrosis (CF) is an autosomal homozygous recessive disorder (*cc*) that causes the production of excessively thick mucus. Using *c* for the CF trait and *C* for not having the CF trait, determine the possible genotypic and phenotypic ratios of offspring produced by a mother with CF and a father who is a carrier for CF. What is the probability that they will have a child who will be a carrier for CF?

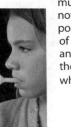

Maternal alleles

Paternal alleles

Maternal alleles

Paternal alleles

13 _____
_____
_____

14 _____
_____
_____

Matching

Match each lettered term with the most closely related description.

a. genotype

b. heterozygous

c. locus

d. autosomes

e. simple inheritance

f. homozygous

g. alleles

h. polygenic inheritance

i. homologous

j. genetics

k. karyotype

l. phenotype

1 Visible characteristics

2 Alternate forms of a gene

3 Refers to the two members of a pair of chromosomes

4 Array of the entire set of chromosomes in a cell

5 An individual's chromosomes and genes

6 Gene's position on a chromosome

7 Two different alleles for the same gene

8 Study of the mechanisms of inheritance

9 Two identical alleles for the same gene

10 Interactions between alleles on several genes

11 Phenotype determined by a single pair of alleles

12 Chromosomes affecting somatic characteristics

1 _____

2 _____

3 _____

4 _____

5 _____

6 _____

7 _____

8 _____

9 _____

10 _____

11 _____

12 _____

Section integration

Using the templates below, draw Punnett squares to answer each question about the following genetic conditions.

13 Tongue-rolling is inherited as a strictly dominant trait. Using *T* for tongue-rolling and *t* for non-tongue-rolling, determine the possible genotypic and phenotypic ratios of offspring born to two heterozygous tongue-rolling parents. What is the probability they will have a child unable to roll his/her tongue?

14 Cystic fibrosis (CF) is an autosomal homozygous recessive disorder (*cc*) that causes the production of excessively thick mucus. Using *c* for the CF trait and *C* for not having the CF trait, determine the possible genotypic and phenotypic ratios of offspring produced by a mother with CF and a father who is a carrier for CF. What is the probability that they will have a child who will be a carrier for CF?

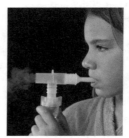

Maternal alleles

Paternal alleles

Maternal alleles

Paternal alleles

13 _____

_____

_____

14 _____

_____

_____

Chapter Review Questions

Indicate whether each statement is true or false.

1 Fertilization typically occurs within the uterus.

2 In the 2 weeks after its development, the yolk sac is the primary nutrient source for the inner cell mass.

3 Dizygotic twins are also called identical twins.

4 Relaxin is a hormone released by the placenta as well as the corpus luteum.

5 There is one umbilical artery and two umbilical veins.

6 The four extra-embryonic membranes are the yolk sac, amnion, allantois, and chorion.

7 The structure that implants in the uterine endometrium is an advanced morula.

8 The health risks associated with oral contraceptives are far greater than the risks associated with pregnancy.

1 _____

2 _____

3 _____

4 _____

5 _____

6 _____

7 _____

8 _____

Multiple choice

Select the correct answer from the list provided.

9 The hormone detected in pregnancy kits is
- ☐ a) relaxin.
- ☐ b) human chorionic gonadotropin (hCG).
- ☐ c) human placental lactogen (hPL).
- ☐ d) gonadotropin-releasing hormone (GnRH).

10 Concerning sex-linked inheritance, X-linked recessive traits
- ☐ a) are more likely to be expressed in females.
- ☐ b) are more likely to be expressed in males.
- ☐ c) are never expressed in females.
- ☐ d) are never expressed in males.

11 Amphimixis is when
- ☐ a) the blastocyst implants into the uterine endometrium.
- ☐ b) a single spermatozoa contacts the oocyte membrane.
- ☐ c) the male pronucleus develops and spindle fibers appear in preparation for cell division.
- ☐ d) the male and female pronuclei fuse.

12 For a given trait T, how would a homozygous dominant genotype be indicated?
- ☐ a) TT
- ☐ b) Tt
- ☐ c) tt
- ☐ d) tT

13 If an allele must be present on both the maternal and paternal chromosomes to affect the phenotype, the allele is said to be
- ☐ a) dominant.
- ☐ b) recessive.
- ☐ c) heterozygous.
- ☐ d) polygenic.

14 Which of the following sex chromosome patterns represents Klinefelter's syndrome?
- ☐ a) YO
- ☐ b) XO
- ☐ c) YYX
- ☐ d) XXY

15 The hormone responsible for milk ejection is
- ☐ a) prolactin.
- ☐ b) estrogen.
- ☐ c) oxytocin.
- ☐ d) progesterone.

16 The phases of labor in the correct order are
- ☐ a) dilation, placental, expulsion.
- ☐ b) placental, dilation, expulsion.
- ☐ c) placental, expulsion, dilation.
- ☐ d) dilation, expulsion, placental.

Short answer

17 Identify the five life stages of postnatal development, and identify the approximate ages for each stage.

18 What is trisomy 21, and what are the risk factors for having a baby with this condition?

CHAPTER 1

Section Reviews

Section 1 Review

1. respiration; **2.** growth and development; **3.** adaptability; **4.** circulation; **5.** excretion; **6.** digestion; **7.** movement; **8.** responsiveness; **9.** Right atrium, Myocardium, Left ventricle, Endocardium, Superior vena cava; **10.** Valve to aorta opens, Valve between left atrium and left ventricle closes, Pressure in left atrium, Electrocardiogram, Heartbeat; **11.** Both keys and messenger molecules have specific three-dimensional shapes, so both can "fit" into and function with their complementary structures (a lock or a receptor protein) only if the shapes match closely enough. Because messenger molecules need not be flat in one dimension (as keys tend to be), they can be very complex in shape, and thus may be able to bind with a variety of complementary receptor proteins. Moreover, although a lock has moving parts, it does not actually change shape, whereas a receptor protein bound by a messenger can change shape, which in turn affects its function. **12.** Larger organisms simply cannot absorb the amount of needed materials or excrete wastes rapidly enough across their body surfaces as well as very small organisms can. Their food must be processed, or digested, before being absorbed, and because the processes of absorption, respiration, and excretion occur in different parts of the organism, an efficient, internal circulation network for their materials is necessary for survival.

Section 2 Review

1. cells; **2.** organs; **3.** organ systems; **4.** epithelial tissue; **5.** external and internal surfaces; **6.** glandular secretions; **7.** connective tissue; **8.** matrix; **9.** protein fibers; **10.** ground substance; **11.** muscle tissue; **12.** movement; **13.** bones of the skeleton; **14.** blood; **15.** materials within digestive tract; **16.** neural

tissue; **17.** neuroglia; **18.** In order from simplest to most complex, the correct levels of organization are: chemical, cellular, tissue, organ, organ system, and organism. **19.** integumentary: protection from environmental hazards, temperature control; **20.** skeletal: provides support, protects soft tissues, stores minerals, forms blood cells; **21.** muscular: provides skeletal movement, guards entrances and exits to body, produces heat, supports skeleton, protects soft tissues; **22.** nervous: directs immediate responses to stimuli, coordinates the activities of other organ systems; **23.** endocrine: controls and regulates growth, development, day-night rhythms, fluid balance, calcium, glucose and water balance, blood cell production, metabolic rate; **24.** cardiovascular: propels and distributes blood, maintains blood pressure, transports gases and nutrients, eliminates wastes, assists in temperature regulation and defense against disease; **25.** lymphatic: transports lymph and lymphocytes, controls immune response and immune cells; **26.** respiratory: filters, warms, and humidifies air; detects smell; conducts air into body; gas exchange between air and blood; **27.** digestive: processing of food and absorption of nutrients, minerals, vitamins, and water; **28.** urinary: eliminates excess water, salts, and waste products; controls blood pH; **29.** reproductive: produces sperm or oocytes, produces hormones, provides the necessary structure and function for sexual intercourse, fetal growth and development, and nourishment of the newborn. **30.** cardiovascular system: blood cells; digestive system: smooth muscle cells; reproductive system: sperm cells (male) and oocytes (female); skeletal system: bone cells (osteocytes); nervous system: nerve cells (neurons). Other cells could be listed for other systems.

Section 3 Review

1. positive feedback; **2.** homeostatic regulation;

3. homeostasis; **4.** sensor; **5.** negative feedback; **6.** negative feedback; **7.** positive feedback; **8.** negative feedback; **9.** positive feedback; **10.** Blood flow to skin increases, sweating increases, body surface cools, and temperature declines. **11.** Blood flow to skin decreases, shivering occurs, body heat is conserved, and temperature rises. **12.** One reason your body temperature may have dropped is that your body may be losing heat faster than it is being produced. (This is more likely to occur on a cool day.) Perhaps hormones have caused a decrease in your metabolic rate, so your body is not producing as much heat as it normally would. Or, you may have an infection that has temporarily reset the set point of the body's "thermostat" to a value higher than normal. The last possibility is the most likely explanation given the circumstances.

Section 4 Review

1. superior; **2.** inferior; **3.** cranial; **4.** caudal; **5.** posterior or dorsal; **6.** anterior or ventral; **7.** lateral; **8.** medial; **9.** proximal; **10.** distal; **11.** proximal; **12.** distal; **13.** thoracic cavity; **14.** mediastinum; **15.** left lung; **16.** trachea, esophagus; **17.** heart; **18.** diaphragm; **19.** abdominopelvic cavity; **20.** peritoneal cavity; **21.** digestive glands and organs; **22.** pelvic cavity; **23.** reproductive organs

Chapter Review Questions

1. right pleural cavity encloses the right lung; **2.** pelvic cavity contains urinary bladder, reproductive organs, and the last portion of the digestive tract; **3.** pericardial cavity encloses the heart; **4.** left pleural cavity encloses the left lung; **5.** diaphragm is a muscular sheet that separates the thoracic cavity and abdominopelvic cavity; **6.** abdominal cavity contains many digestive glands and organs enclosed by the peritoneum; **7.** c; **8.** e; **9.** k; **10.** b; **11.** j; **12.** h; **13.** a; **14.** i; **15.** n; **16.** d; **17.** f; **18.** m; **19.** g; **20.** l; **21.** b; **22.** d; **23.** b; **24.** b; **25.** c; **26.** d; **27.** c; **28.** b; **29.** Anatomy is

the study of structure. Physiology is the study of function. **30.** The three basic principles of the cell theory are: 1. Cells are the structural building blocks of all plants and animals. 2. Cells are produced by the divisions of pre-existing cells. 3. Cells are the smallest structural units that perform all vital functions. **31.** The heart is enclosed by the pericardial cavity; the small intestine is enclosed by the peritoneum within the abdominal cavity; the large intestine is enclosed by the peritoneum within the abdominal cavity, but with the last portion in the pelvic cavity (infraperitoneal); the lungs are enclosed by the pleural cavities; the kidneys are retroperitoneal. **32.** The four main tissue types are epithelial tissue, connective tissue, muscle tissue, and neural tissue. Module 1.7 identifies a comprehensive list of where these tissues are found in the body. **33.** Calcitonin is released when calcium levels are elevated. This hormone should bring about a decrease in blood calcium levels, thus decreasing the stimulus for its release. **34.** A stroke causes damage to the brain, the organ responsible for controlling both voluntary and autonomic activities. Therefore, a patient could lose control of voluntary activities such as walking or speech. Autonomic activities such as bladder control could also be lost.

CHAPTER 2

Section Reviews

Section 1 Review

1. f; **2.** d; **3.** k; **4.** a; **5.** l; **6.** h; **7.** i; **8.** j; **9.** c; **10.** e; **11.** g; **12.** b; **13.** 2; **14.** 4; **15.** 1; **16.** 0; **17.** 6; **18.** 12; **19.** 7; **20.** 7; **21.** 20; **22.** 20; **23.** molecule; **24.** compound; **25.** molecule; **26.** compound; **27.** The outer energy level of inert elements is filled with electrons, whereas the outer energy level of reactive elements is not filled with electrons. Atoms with unfilled outer energy levels will react with other atoms. Atoms with filled outer energy levels will not react with other atoms. **28.** Both polar and nonpolar molecules are held together by covalent bonds. However, in a polar molecule the electrons are not shared equally, so it carries small, or partial, positive and negative charges on its surface; in a nonpolar molecule the electrons are shared equally, so it is electrically neutral. **29.** Both covalent bonds and ionic bonds bind atoms together, but covalent bonds involve the sharing of electrons between atoms, whereas ionic bonds involve the electrical attraction of oppositely charged atoms (ions).

Section 2 Review

1. h; **2.** g; **3.** e; **4.** f; **5.** d; **6.** c; **7.** a; **8.** b; **9.** H_2; **10.** 2 H; **11.** 6 H_2O; **12.** $C_{12}H_{22}O_{11}$; **13.** $C_6H_{12}O_6 + 6\ O_2 \rightarrow 6\ CO_2 + 6\ H_2O$; **14.** hydrolysis reaction; **15.** dehydration synthesis reaction; **16.** A decreased amount of enzyme at the second step would limit the amount of the intermediate products in the next two steps. This would cause a decrease in the amount of the final product.

Section 3 Review

1. e; **2.** h; **3.** i; **4.** d; **5.** a; **6.** j; **7.** c; **8.** g; **9.** f; **10.** b; **11.** effective lubrication (as between bony surfaces in a joint); **12.** reactivity (participates in chemical reactions); **13.** high heat capacity (readily absorbs and retains heat); **14.** solubility (is a solvent for many substances); **15.** acidic; **16.** neutral; **17.** alkaline; **18.** The pH 3 solution is 1000 times more acidic than the pH 6 solution—it contains a one-thousandfold (10^3) increase in the concentration of hydrogen ions (H^+). **19.** Three negative effects of abnormal fluctuations in pH are cell and tissue damage (due to broken bonds), changes in the shapes of proteins, and altered cellular functions. **20.** Table salt dissociates (dissolves) in pure water but because it does not release either hydrogen ions (H^+) or hydroxide ions (OH^-), no change in pH occurs.

Section 4 Review

1. carbohydrates; **2.** polysaccha-rides; **3.** disaccharides; **4.** monosaccharides; **5.** lipids;

6. fatty acids; **7.** glycerol; **8.** proteins; **9.** amino acids; **10.** nucleic acids; **11.** RNA; **12.** DNA; **13.** nucleotides; **14.** ATP; **15.** phosphate groups; **16.** polysaccharide, polyunsaturated, polypeptide; **17.** triglyceride; **18.** disaccharide, diglyceride, dipeptide; **19.** glycogen, glycolipids; **20.** g; **21.** f; **22.** c; **23.** h; **24.** d; **25.** e; **26.** b; **27.** j; **28.** k; **29.** i; **30.** a

Chapter Review Questions

1. c; **2.** c; **3.** b; **4.** e; **5.** c; **6.** a; **7.** c; **8.** b; **9.** d; **10.** a; **11.** b; **12.** d; **13.** c; **14.** b; **15.** d; **16.** a; **17.** b; **18.** d; **19.** protons, neutrons, and electrons; **20.** carbohydrates, lipids, proteins, and nucleic acids; **21.** Lipids perform many functions in the body including: energy reserve, insulation and heat conservation, organ protection, chemical messengers, structural components of cell membranes, and digestive secretions. **22.** Proteins are long chains of amino acids bound together by peptide bonds. Progressive folding and pleating of the chain into more complex shapes modifies the primary linear arrangement of amino acids. The increasing levels of complexity are primary, secondary, tertiary, and quaternary structures. **23. (a)** DNA: deoxyribose, phosphate, and nitrogenous bases (A, T, C, G); **(b)** RNA: ribose, phosphate, and nitrogenous bases (A, U, C, G); **24.** Enzymes are specialized protein catalysts that lower the activation energy for chemical reactions. Enzymes speed up chemical reactions but are not used up or changed in the process. **25.** A salt is an ionic compound consisting of any cations other than hydrogen ions and any anions other than hydroxide ions. Acids dissociate and release hydrogen ions, whereas bases remove hydrogen ions from solution (usually by releasing hydroxide ions). **26.** Nonpolar covalent bonds involve an equal sharing of electrons. Polar covalent bonds involve an unequal sharing of

electrons. Ionic bonds result from the attraction of oppositely charged ions. (Ions are atoms which have either lost or gained electrons.) **27.** The molecule is a nucleic acid. Carbohydrates and lipids do not contain nitrogen. Although both proteins and nucleic acids contain nitrogen, only nucleic acids normally contain phosphorus. **28.** The insect can walk across the surface of the pond because its small mass is not sufficient to break the surface tension created by the hydrogen bonds between the water molecules. **29.** All of the foods and drink that the student consumed have a pH below 7 and are therefore acidic. These acidic foods, in conjunction with the hydrochloric acid in his stomach necessary for digestion, are likely the cause of his upset stomach. Consuming foods that are slightly alkaline could buffer his stomach contents and relieve his symptoms.
30. (a)

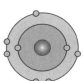

Oxygen atom

(b) Two more electrons can fit into the outermost energy level of an oxygen atom.

CHAPTER 3

Section Reviews

Section 1 Review

1. glycolysis; **2.** aerobic (metabolism); **3.** microvilli; **4.** lysosome; **5.** microvilli: increase surface area to facilitate absorption of extracellular materials; **6.** Golgi apparatus: stores, alters, and packages newly synthesized proteins; **7.** lysosome: intracellular removal of pathogens or damaged organelles; **8.** mitochondrion: produces 95 percent of the ATP required by the cell; **9.** peroxisome: neutralizes toxic

compounds; **10.** nucleus: controls metabolism, stores and processes genetic information, controls protein synthesis; **11.** rough endoplasmic reticulum: has ribosomes bound to the membranes, modifies and packages newly synthesized proteins; **12.** ribosomes: protein synthesis; **13.** cytoskeleton: provides strength and support, enables movement of cellular structures and materials; **14.** Similar to the role of a plasma membrane around a cell, an organelle membrane physically isolates the organelle's contents from the cytosol, regulates exchange with the cytosol, and provides structural support.

Section 2 Review

1. d; **2.** h; **3.** l; **4.** a; **5.** k; **6.** n; **7.** m; **8.** b; **9.** j; **10.** e; **11.** i; **12.** c; **13.** g; **14.** f; **15.** AUG/UUU/UGU/GCC/GCC/UUA; **16.** UAC/AAA/ACA/CGG/CGG/AAU; **17.** Methionine-Phenylalanine-Cysteine-Alanine-Alanine-Leucine; **18.** The nucleus contains the information for synthesizing proteins in the nucleotide sequence of its DNA. Changes in the extracellular fluid can affect cells through the binding of molecules to plasma membrane receptors or by the diffusion of molecules through membrane channels. Such stimuli may result in alterations of genetic activity in the nucleus. These alterations may change biochemical processes and metabolic pathways through the synthesis of additional, fewer, or different enzymes. Altered genetic activity may also change the physical structure of the cell by synthesizing additional, fewer, or different structural proteins.

Section 3 Review

1. diffusion; **2.** facilitated diffusion; **3.** molecular size; **4.** net diffusion of water; **5.** active transport; **6.** specificity; **7.** vesicular transport; **8.** exocytosis; **9.** pinocytosis; **10.** "cell eating"; **11.** diffusion; **12.** neither; **13.** osmosis; **14.** diffusion; **15.** osmosis

Section 4 Review

1. somatic cells; **2.** G_1 phase; **3.** G_2 phase; **4.** DNA replication; **5.** mitosis; **6.** metaphase; **7.** telophase; **8.** cytokinesis; **9.** telophase; **10.** prophase; **11.** centromere; **12.** A cell that undergoes repeated rounds of the cell cycle without cytokinesis could result in a large, multinucleated cell.

Chapter Review Questions

1. b; **2.** c; **3.** b; **4.** b; **5.** a; **6.** b; **7.** a; **8.** b; **9.** d; **10.** b; **11.** c; **12.** c; **13.** anchoring proteins, recognition proteins, receptor proteins, carrier proteins, and channels; **14.** Mitosis specifically refers to the division and duplication of the cell's nucleus. Cytokinesis is the division of the cytoplasm into two distinct new cells. **15.** Diffusion is the movement of solutes by concentration differences. Osmosis is the net diffusion of water across a membrane. **16.** Mitochondria contain their own DNA called mtDNA. It codes for small numbers of RNA and polypeptide molecules. The polypeptides are used in enzymes required for energy production. **17.** The nonmembranous organelles are the cytoskeleton, microvilli, centrioles, cilia, flagella, and ribosomes. The membranous organelles are the mitochondria, nucleus, endoplasmic reticulum, Golgi apparatus, lysosomes, and peroxisomes. **18.** Prophase: chromosomes coil forming visible chromosomes, each copy called a chromatid. Metaphase: chromatids move to the metaphase plate. Anaphase: centromere of each chromatid pair splits and the chromatids separate. Telophase: each new cell prepares to return to interphase, nuclear membranes re-form, nuclei enlarge, and chromosomes uncoil; **19.** If a cell had microvilli on its plasma membrane it is likely to be actively engaged in absorbing materials from the extracellular fluid. **20.** The cell would swell up like a balloon and may eventually burst, releasing its contents. This event is called hemolysis. **21.** e, b, a, g, f,

c, d; **22.** Phagocytosis begins when cytoplasmic extensions called pseudopodia surround targeted material. The pseudopodia fuse to form a phagosome containing the targeted material. This vesicle fuses with lysosomes. Lysosomal enzymes digest the targeted material. Nutrients are released from the vesicle, and the residue is ejected from the cell through exocytosis. **23.** All somatic cells contain 46 chromosomes. Since mitosis produces two identical nuclei, the resulting cells will each have 46 chromosomes. Meiosis produces sex cells (sperm or oocytes) containing 23 chromosomes, which can unite to form a new somatic cell of 46 chromosomes. **24.** Lipid molecules such as steroid hormones are lipid soluble and therefore easily diffuse across the lipid bilayer of the plasma membrane. **25.** Malignant tumors divide rapidly and release chemicals that stimulate the growth of blood vessels in a process called angiogenesis. The availability of additional nutrients from these new vessels accelerates tumor growth and metastasis.

CHAPTER 4

Section Reviews

Section 1 Review

1. simple squamous epithelium; **2.** simple cuboidal epithelium; **3.** simple columnar epithelium; **4.** stratified squamous epithelium; **5.** stratified cuboidal epithelium; **6.** stratified columnar epithelium; **7.** mucous cells; **8.** mucin; **9.** mucus; **10.** ducts; **11.** epithelial surfaces; **12.** exocrine glands; **13.** merocrine secretion; **14.** apocrine secretion; **15.** holocrine secretion; **16.** interstitial fluid; **17.** endocrine glands; **18.** avascular; **19.** alveolar (acinar) gland; **20.** transitional epithelium; **21.** occluding junction; **22.** basal lamina; **23.** simple gland; **24.** mesothelium (simple squamous epithelium); **25.** pseudostratified columnar epithelium; **26.** urinary

bladder, ureters, urine-collecting chambers in the kidney; **27.** stratified squamous epithelium; **28.** simple columnar epithelium; **29.** lining of the peritoneum and pericardium, exchange surfaces (alveoli) within the lungs; **30.** lining of exocrine glands and ducts, kidney tubules; **31.** stratified cuboidal epithelium

Section 2 Review

1. loose connective tissue; **2.** adipose; **3.** regular; **4.** tendons; **5.** ligaments; **6.** fluid connective tissue; **7.** blood; **8.** hyaline; **9.** chondrocytes in lacunae; **10.** bone; **11.** perichondrium, periosteum, peritoneum, pericardium; **12.** periosteum, osteocytes, osteon; **13.** chondrocyte, perichondrium; **14.** interstitial growth; **15.** lacunae; **16.** chondrocyte; **17.** osseous tissue; **18.** fibrocartilage; **19.** adipocytes; **20.** synovial membrane; **21.** cutaneous membrane; **22.** perichondrium

Section 3 Review

1. cardiac; **2.** smooth; **3.** nonstriated; **4.** multinucleate; **5.** cell body; **6.** dendrites; **7.** neuroglia; **8.** maintain physical structure of neural tissue; **9.** repair neural tissue framework after injury; **10.** perform phagocytosis; **11.** provide nutrients to neurons; **12.** regulate the composition of interstitial fluid surrounding neurons; **13.** axon; **14.** intercalated disc; **15.** neuroglia; **16.** skeletal muscle tissue; **17.** smooth muscle tissue; **18.** regeneration; **19.** inflammation; **20.** Increased blood flow and blood vessel permeability enhance the delivery of oxygen and nutrients and the migration of additional phagocytes into the area, and the removal of toxins and waste products from the area.

Chapter Review Questions

1. hyaline cartilage; **2.** elastic cartilage; **3.** fibrocartilage; **4.** cardiac muscle tissue; **5.** smooth muscle tissue; **6.** skeletal muscle tissue; **7.** bone or osseous tissue; **8.** adipose tissue; **9.** dense regular

connective tissue; **10.** reticular tissue; **11.** areolar tissue; **12.** fluid connective tissues (blood and lymph); **13.** c; **14.** b; **15.** c; **16.** a; **17.** d; **18.** b; **19.** b; **20.** a; **21.** b; **22.** d; **23.** The skin and the lining of the mouth and throat are areas regularly exposed to severe mechanical or chemical stresses. The superficial cells, therefore, are continually worn away due to these stressors and must be replaced by cells in deeper layers. Stratified squamous epithelium contains a series of layers that allow for deeper cells to replace the lost superficial cells. **24.** Endocrine glands secrete hormones onto the surface of the gland or directly into the surrounding fluid. Exocrine glands secrete directly into ducts. **25.** Neural tissue contains (1) neurons, which transmit electrical impulses, and (2) neuroglia, which protect, support, and repair neural tissue and maintain the nutrient supply to neurons. **26.** Normally the extensive interlocking connections between the epithelial skin cells protect from infection by blocking pathogen access. After a severe skin burn or abrasion, this mechanism can no longer provide protection and pathogens easily enter the deeper tissues, resulting in an infection. **27.** Underneath a light microscope cardiac muscle tissue would demonstrate branched cells, striations, a single nucleus, and intercalated discs. **28.** Skeletal muscle tissue is made up of densely packed fibers running parallel that demonstrate striations, but because muscle fibers are composed of cells, they also have many visible nuclei. Jason is probably looking at a tendon (dense regular connective tissue). The small nuclei would be those of fibroblasts. **29.** The skin in the injured area will become red, warm, swollen, and painful. These changes occur as a result of inflammation, the body's first response to injury. Injury to the epithelium and underlying connective tissue will trigger the release of chemicals such as histamine and heparin from mast cells in the area. These chemicals, in turn, initiate the changes identified above.

CHAPTER 5

Section Reviews

Section 1 Review
1. accessory structures;
2. epidermis; 3. granulosum;
4. papillary layer; 5. nerves;
6. reticular layer; 7. collagen;
8. hypodermis; 9. connective;
10. fat; 11. dermis: the connective tissue layer beneath the epidermis; 12. epidermis: the protective epithelium covering the surface of the skin; 13. papillary layer: vascularized areolar tissue containing capillaries, lymphatic vessels, and sensory neurons that supply the skin surface; 14. reticular layer: interwoven meshwork of dense irregular connective tissue containing collagen fibers and elastic fibers; 15. hypodermis (subcutaneous layer or superficial fascia): layer of loose connective tissue below the dermis;
16. Malignant melanoma is often fatal because melanocytes are located close to the dermal layer, so if they become malignant, they can easily metastasize through the blood vessels and lymphatic vessels in nearby connective tissues; 17. The firefighter's comment that his burns are not painful should concern the doctors because it indicates that these are third-degree burns. This type of burn is full-thickness and can destroy the sensory neurons, which is why the firefighter could not detect pain, despite being seriously burned.

Section 2 Review
1. free edge; 2. lateral nail fold;
3. nail body; 4. lunula; 5. proximal nail fold; 6. eponychium;
7. eponychium; 8. proximal nail fold; 9. nail root; 10. lunula;
11. nail body; 12. hyponychium;
13. phalanx; 14. dermis;
15. epidermis; 16. hair shaft;
17. sebaceous gland; 18. arrector pili muscle; 19. connective tissue

sheath of hair bulb; 20. root hair plexus; 21. h; 22. c; 23. e; 24. g;
25. i; 26. b; 27. d; 28. a; 29. j;
30. f; 31. The chemicals in hair dyes break the protective covering of the cortex, allowing the dyes to stain the medulla of the shaft. This is not permanent because the cortex remains damaged, allowing shampoo and UV rays from the sun to enter the medulla and affect the color. Also, the viable portion of the hair remains unaffected, so that when the shaft is replaced, the color or any change in curl will be lost.

Chapter Review Questions

1. stratum corneum; 2. stratum lucidum; 3. stratum granulosum;
4. stratum spinosum; 5. stratum basale; 6. false; 7. true; 8. false;
9. false; 10. true; 11. true;
12. false; 13. true; 14. b; 15. b;
16. b; 17. d; 18. a; 19. b; 20. c;
21. a; 22. epidermis, dermis;
23. subcutaneous; 24. Apocrine;
25. basal cell carcinoma;
26. melanin; 27. Epidermal cell division occurs in the stratum basale. 28. These smooth muscles cause hairs to stand erect when stimulated. 29. Variations in hair color are due to differences in the pigment produced by the melanocytes in the hair papilla. With age, pigment production decreases, and hair color lightens. White hair is due to the combination of no pigment and air bubbles in the hair shaft medulla. 30. A lack of vitamin D_3 can result in rickets in children. In adults, it can lead to decreased bone density, and a greater risk for bone fractures. 31. Compared to the thin skin of the rest of the body, the thick skin of the palms of the hands has a much thicker stratum corneum, and also contains a stratum lucidum. The heat from the campfire, therefore, has less tissue to penetrate on the thin skin of your face before reaching the sensory neurons.
32. A cut parallel to the cleavage lines will usually remain closed and heal with little scarring. A cut at right angles to a cleavage line will be pulled open as severed

elastic fibers recoil and will result in greater scarring. 33. Using the rule of nines, the right leg is 19 percent of surface area, the right arm is 9 percent of surface area, and the back of the trunk is 18 percent of body area. Summing these numbers estimates that this patient has burned 46 percent of her body.

CHAPTER 6

Section Reviews

Section 1 Review
1. intramembranous ossification;
2. collagen; 3. osteocytes;
4. lacunae; 5. hyaline cartilage;
6. periosteum; 7. compact bone;
8. irregular bones; 9. epiphyses;
10. fossa; 11. medullary cavity;
12. trabeculae; 13. osteoclasts;
14. sesamoid bones; 15. ossification or osteogenesis; 16. osteon;
17. appositional growth;
18. endochondral ossification;
19. The fracture might have damaged the epiphyseal cartilage in Rebecca's right leg. Even though the bone healed properly, the damaged leg did not produce as much cartilage as did the undamaged leg. The result would be a shorter bone on the side of the injury.

Section 2 Review
1. calcitonin; 2. ↓ Ca^{2+} concentration in blood; 3. ↓ Ca^{2+} level; 4. parathyroid glands;
5. ↑ Ca^{2+} concentration in blood;
6. release of stored Ca^{2+} from bone; 7. homeostasis; 8. spiral fracture; 9. transverse fracture;
10. greenstick fracture;
11. comminuted fracture;
12. compression fracture;
13. Colles fracture

Chapter Review Questions

1. epiphysis; 2. metaphysis;
3. diaphysis; 4. epiphysis;
5. spongy bone or cancellous bone or trabecular bone; 6. compact bone; 7. medullary cavity; 8. true;
9. false; 10. true; 11. true;
12. false; 13. true; 14. false;
15. true; 16. b; 17. c; 18. a; 19. b;

20. d; 21. c; 22. a; 23. b; 24. c;
25. 80, 126; 26. Sesamoid;
27. sinus; 28. osteon or Haversian system; 29. Osteoclasts;
30. (1) support, (2) storage of minerals and lipids, (3) blood cell production, (4) protection, (5) leverage; 31. The twisting forces of a pirouette are likely to cause a spiral fracture. 32. Pituitary growth failure causes reduced epiphyseal cartilage activity and therefore abnormally short bones. This is rare because children can be treated with synthetic growth hormone. Achondroplasia is caused by reduced epiphyseal activity resulting in short, stocky limbs. The trunk, however, is of normal size. 33. In intramembranous ossification, bone replaces mesenchymal cells or fibrous connective tissue. In endochondral ossification, bone replaces a cartilage model. 34. An epiphyseal fracture is of particular concern because the cartilage can stop growing as it heals. This could result in the fractured limb being shorter than the opposite limb.
35. Since the osteons of compact bone run parallel to the long axis of the shaft, impacts perpendicular to the length of the bone are more likely to cause a fracture than stresses parallel to the length of the bone. 36. Gigantism is overproduction of growth hormone (GH) before puberty. People with gigantism can be very tall, exceeding 2.7 m (8 ft 11 in.). In acromegaly, GH rises after puberty, so the person does not grow taller, but the bones become thicker. Facial contours change in a characteristic manner.

CHAPTER 7

Section Reviews

Section 1 Review
1. frontal; 2. sphenoid;
3. zygomatic; 4. ethmoid;
5. lacrimal; 6. palatine; 7. maxilla;
8. sphenoidal fontanelle;
9. squamous suture; 10. lambdoid suture; 11. mastoid fontanelle;
12. anterior fontanelle;
13. sagittal suture; 14. occipital

fontanelle; **15.** Region: thoracic; **16.** Characteristics: found in chest, heart-shaped body, smaller vertebral foramen, long slender spinous process that points inferiorly, all but two have facets for rib articulations; **17.** Region: cervical; **18.** Characteristics: found in neck, small oval body, large vertebral foramen, bifid spinous process, transverse foramina; **19.** Region: lumbar; **20.** Characteristics: found in inferior back, massive vertebral body, smallest vertebral foramen, spinous process blunt and projects posteriorly, no articular facets for ribs or transverse foramina.

Section 2 Review

1. clavicle; **2.** scapula; **3.** humerus; **4.** radius; **5.** ulna; **6.** carpal bones; **7.** metacarpal bones; **8.** phalanges; **9.** hip bone (coxal bone); **10.** femur; **11.** patella; **12.** tibia; **13.** fibula; **14.** tarsal bones; **15.** metatarsal bones; **16.** phalanges; **17.** Sex: female; **18.** Differences: smoother, lighter, less prominent markings, enlarged pelvic outlet, pubic angle greater than 100°, less curvature of sacrum and coccyx, ilia project more laterally; **19.** Sex: male; **20.** Differences: rougher, heavier, more prominent markings, smaller pelvic outlet, pubic angle less than 100°, more curvature of sacrum and coccyx, ilia project more superiorly.

Chapter Review Questions

1. occipital bone; **2.** parietal bone; **3.** frontal bone; **4.** temporal bone; **5.** sphenoid **6.** ethmoid; **7.** vomer; **8.** mandible; **9.** lacrimal bone; **10.** nasal bone; **11.** zygomatic bone; **12.** maxilla; **13.** true; **14.** false; **15.** false; **16.** true; **17.** c; **18.** c; **19.** b; **20.** d; **21.** b; **22.** b; **23.** b; **24.** a; **25.** Fontanelles, which are fibrous connections between cranial bones in the infant, permit the skull to distort without damage during delivery, helping to ease the infant through the birth canal. **26.** Movement of the ribs affects the width and depth of the thoracic cage, increasing or decreasing its

volume accordingly. This change in volume assists in breathing by increasing and decreasing the pressure inside the thoracic cavity. **27.** The three bones that fuse to form the hip bone (or coxal bone) are the ilium, ischium, and pubis. They meet at the acetabulum. **28.** Primary curves develop before birth, and the secondary curves develop after birth. The thoracic curve and sacral curves are primary curves. The cervical curve is a secondary curve that forms as an infant begins to balance the weight of the head. The lumbar curve is a secondary curve that develops with the ability to stand. **29.** Arches assist with transferring the weight of the body to the feet and eventually to the ground. The longitudinal arch runs from the calcaneus to the distal metatarsals. The transverse arch runs perpendicular to the longitudinal arch and is the result of the change in the degree of longitudinal arch curvature from the medial border to the lateral border of the foot.

CHAPTER 8

Section Reviews

Section 1 Review

1. medullary cavity; **2.** spongy bone; **3.** periosteum; **4.** synovial membrane; **5.** articular cartilage; **6.** joint cavity (containing synovial fluid); **7.** joint capsule; **8.** compact bone; **9.** flexion; **10.** extension; **11.** hyperextension; **12.** flexion; **13.** hyperextension; **14.** abduction; **15.** adduction; **16.** head rotation; **17.** pronation; **18.** abduction; **19.** adduction; **20.** opposition; **21.** e; **22.** d; **23.** f; **24.** g; **25.** b; **26.** c; **27.** h; **28.** a

Section 2 Review

1. coracoclavicular ligaments; **2.** acromioclavicular ligament; **3.** tendon of supraspinatus muscle; **4.** acromion; **5.** articular capsule; **6.** subdeltoid bursa; **7.** synovial membrane; **8.** humerus; **9.** clavicle;

10. coracoacromial ligament; **11.** coracoid process; **12.** scapula; **13.** articular cartilages; **14.** joint cavity; **15.** glenoid labrum; **16.** patellar surface of femur; **17.** fibular collateral ligament or lateral collateral ligament; **18.** lateral condyle; **19.** lateral meniscus; **20.** tibia; **21.** fibula; **22.** posterior cruciate ligament (PCL); **23.** medial condyle; **24.** tibial collateral ligament or medial collateral ligament; **25.** medial meniscus; **26.** anterior cruciate ligament (ACL); **27.** b; **28.** e; **29.** h; **30.** g; **31.** c; **32.** a; **33.** f; **34.** d; **35.** The sternoclavicular joints are the only joints between the pectoral girdles and the axial skeleton. The sacroiliac joints are the joints between the pelvic girdle and the axial skeleton.

Chapter Review Questions

1. true; **2.** false; **3.** false; **4.** true; **5.** true; **6.** false; **7.** d; **8.** c; **9.** c; **10.** d; **11.** d; **12.** c; **13.** b; **14.** b; **15.** b; **16.** b; **17.** d; **18.** a; **19.** b; **20.** c; **21.** In a bulging disc, the nucleus pulposus does not extrude. In a herniated disc, the nucleus pulposus breaks through the anulus fibrosus. **22.** Articular cartilage lacks a perichondrium, and its matrix contains more water than does the matrix of other cartilages. **23.** (1) gliding joint: sternoclavicular joint; (2) hinge joint: elbow joint; (3) pivot joint: proximal radioulnar joint; (4) condylar joint: radiocarpal joints; (5) saddle joint: first carpometacarpal joint; (6) ball-and-socket joint: shoulder joint; **24.** Menisci may subdivide a synovial cavity, channel the flow of synovial fluid, or allow for variations in the shapes of articular surfaces to assist with joint stability and cushioning. **25.** A loss of bone mass as a result of aging is called osteopenia. When the reduction of bone mass is sufficient to compromise normal function, the condition is called osteoporosis.

CHAPTER 9

Section Reviews

Section 1 Review

1. mitochondrion; **2.** sarcolemma; **3.** myofibril; **4.** thin filament; **5.** thick filament; **6.** triad; **7.** sarcoplasmic reticulum; **8.** T tubule; **9.** terminal cisterna; **10.** sarcoplasm; **11.** myofibril; **12.** I band; **13.** A band; **14.** H band; **15.** Z line; **16.** titin; **17.** zone of overlap; **18.** M line; **19.** thin filament; **20.** thick filament; **21.** sarcomere; **22.** skeletal muscle; **23.** muscle fascicle; **24.** muscle fiber; **25.** myofibril; **26.** myofilament; **27.** sarcomere

Section 2 Review

1. fatty acids; **2.** O_2; **3.** glucose; **4.** glycogen; **5.** CP; **6.** creatine; **7.** b; **8.** c; **9.** a; **10.** d; **11.** large; **12.** small; **13.** intermediate; **14.** white; **15.** pink; **16.** low; **17.** high; **18.** dense; **19.** intermediate; **20.** few; **21.** many; **22.** intermediate; **23.** rapid; **24.** medium; **25.** fast; **26.** slow; **27.** fast; **28.** low; **29.** high; **30.** low; **31.** high

Chapter Review Questions

1. true; **2.** false; **3.** true; **4.** false; **5.** b; **6.** g; **7.** i; **8.** c; **9.** a; **10.** h; **11.** j; **12.** f; **13.** e; **14.** d; **15.** d; **16.** b; **17.** a; **18.** b; **19.** d; **20.** a; **21.** b; **22.** c; **23.** a; **24.** d; **25.** The T tubules conduct action potentials into the interior of the cell. **26.** When contracting to lift the coffee cup, the muscles of elbow joint flexion are recruiting few motor units. The greater tension required for curling a dumbbell would be achieved by recruitment of more motor units including motor units of more powerful muscle fibers. **27.** Throughout the recovery period, oxygen demand remains above normal resting levels as the liver absorbs and recycles the lactate released by muscle fibers during intense exercise. The liver converts the lactate to glucose, which is released into the bloodstream. The transport of lactate to the liver and of glucose back to muscle cells is called the Cori cycle. The additional oxygen consumed by the liver for glucose synthesis is called the oxygen debt, or excess postexercise oxygen consumption. The muscle fibers use the glucose to restore ATP, creatine phosphate, and glycogen concentrations to pre-exertion levels. **28.** Aerobic metabolism and glycolysis generate ATP from glucose in muscle cells. **29.** When a muscle experiences repeated, exhaustive stimulation, as in exercise, muscle fibers develop more mitochondria, a higher concentration of glycolytic enzymes, larger glycogen reserves, and more myofibrils. Each myofibril contains more thick and thin filaments. The net effect is hypertrophy, or enlargement of the stimulated muscle.

CHAPTER 10

Section Reviews

Section 1 Review

1. unipennate; **2.** convergent; **3.** bipennate; **4.** circular or sphincter; **5.** multipennate; **6.** sternocleidomastoid; **7.** deltoid; **8.** biceps brachii; **9.** external oblique; **10.** pronator teres; **11.** brachioradialis; **12.** flexor carpi radialis; **13.** rectus femoris; **14.** vastus lateralis; **15.** vastus medialis; **16.** gastrocnemius; **17.** soleus; **18.** pectoralis major; **19.** rectus abdominis; **20.** iliopsoas; **21.** tensor fascia latae; **22.** gracilis; **23.** sartorius; **24.** tibialis anterior; **25.** extensor digitorum longus

Section 2 Review

1. occipitofrontalis (frontal belly); **2.** temporalis; **3.** orbicularis oculi; **4.** levator labii superioris; **5.** zygomaticus minor; **6.** zygomaticus major; **7.** buccinator; **8.** orbicularis oris; **9.** risorius; **10.** depressor labii inferioris; **11.** depressor anguli oris; **12.** masseter; **13.** mylohyoid; **14.** digastric; **15.** geniohyoid;

16. omohyoid; **17.** stylohyoid; **18.** thyrohyoid; **19.** sternothyroid; **20.** sternohyoid; **21.** sternocleidomastoid

Section 3 Review

1. triceps brachii, long head; **2.** anconeus; **3.** extensor carpi ulnaris; **4.** extensor carpi radialis longus; **5.** extensor digitorum; **6.** flexor carpi ulnaris; **7.** gluteus medius; **8.** tensor fasciae latae; **9.** gluteus maximus; **10.** adductor magnus; **11.** gracilis; **12.** biceps femoris; **13.** semitendinosus; **14.** semimembranosus; **15.** sartorius; **16.** popliteus; **17.** gastrocnemius; **18.** tibialis anterior; **19.** fibularis longus; **20.** soleus; **21.** extensor digitorum longus; **22.** fibularis brevis; **23.** superior extensor retinaculum; **24.** inferior extensor retinaculum; **25.** calcaneal tendon

Chapter Review Questions

1. second-class lever; **2.** first-class lever; **3.** third-class lever; **4.** true; **5.** false; **6.** true; **7.** true; **8.** false; **9.** j; **10.** h; **11.** f; **12.** a; **13.** g; **14.** b; **15.** e; **16.** c; **17.** d; **18.** i; **19.** b; **20.** b; **21.** c; **22.** a; **23.** a; **24.** c; **25.** d; **26.** a; **27.** c; **28.** b; **29.** The muscles of the pelvic floor support the organs of the pelvic cavity, flex the coccygeal joints, and control the movement of materials through the anus and urethra. **30.** The muscles of the rotator cuff are supraspinatus, infraspinatus, teres minor, and subscapularis. **31.** The muscles of the quadriceps muscle group are rectus femoris, vastus intermedius, vastus medialis, and vastus lateralis. These muscles produce extension at the knee. Rectus femoris also produces flexion at the hip.

CHAPTER 11

Section Reviews

Section 1 Review

1. dendrite; **2.** Nissl bodies; **3.** mitochondrion; **4.** nucleus; **5.** nucleolus; **6.** cell body;

7. axon hillock; **8.** initial segment; **9.** axolemma; **10.** axon; **11.** telodendrion; **12.** axon terminal; **13.** multipolar; **14.** unipolar; **15.** anaxonic; **16.** bipolar; **17.** neuron, neuroglia, neurofilaments, neurofibrils, neurotubules, neurilemma; **18.** dendrite, dendritic spines, telodendria, oligodendrocytes; **19.** efferent fibers; **20.** afferent fibers

Section 2 Review

1. action potential; **2.** electrical synapse; **3.** resting potential; **4.** gated channels; **5.** cholinergic synapses; **6.** hyperpolarization; **7.** local current; **8.** depolarization; **9.** acetylcholine (ACh); **10.** calcium ions (Ca^{2+}); **11.** synaptic vesicle; **12.** acetylcholinesterase (AChE); **13.** ACh receptor; **14.** sodium ions (Na^+); **15.** An action potential depolarizes the axon terminal. **16.** Calcium ions enter the cytosol of the axon terminal. **17.** ACh is released through exocytosis. **18.** ACh binds to sodium channel receptors on the postsynaptic membrane, producing a graded depolarization. **19.** The depolarization ends as ACh is broken down into acetate and choline by AChE. **20.** The axon terminal reabsorbs choline from the synaptic cleft and uses it to synthesize new molecules of ACh. **21.** In myelinated fibers, saltatory propagation transmits nerve impulses to the neuromuscular junctions rapidly enough to initiate muscle contractions and promote normal movements. In axons that have become demyelinated, nerve impulses cannot be propagated, so the muscles are not stimulated to contract. Eventually, the muscles atrophy from lack of stimulation (a condition termed disuse atrophy).

Chapter Review Questions

1. ependymal cell; **2.** astrocyte; **3.** node (node of Ranvier); **4.** axon; **5.** oligodendrocyte; **6.** myelinated axon; **7.** neuron cell body; **8.** microglia; **9.** false; **10.** true; **11.** false; **12.** true; **13.** true;

14. c; **15.** e; **16.** a; **17.** b; **18.** f; **19.** g; **20.** h; **21.** d; **22.** c; **23.** b; **24.** b; **25.** c; **26.** d; **27.** a; **28.** b; **29.** The central nervous system (CNS) is composed of the brain and spinal cord. The peripheral nervous system (PNS) is made up of all the neural tissue outside the CNS and is divided into the sensory and motor divisions. **30.** The three functional classes of neurons in the nervous system are sensory neurons, interneurons, and motor neurons. Sensory neurons transmit impulses from the PNS to the CNS. Interneurons analyze sensory inputs and coordinate motor outputs. Motor neurons transmit impulses from the CNS to the PNS. **31.** In continuous propagation, which occurs in unmyelinated axons, an action potential appears to move across the membrane surface in a series of tiny steps. In saltatory propagation, which occurs in myelinated axons, only the nodes can respond to a depolarizing stimulus. Saltatory propagation is much faster than continuous propagation. **32.** Localized changes in membrane potential that cannot spread far from the site of stimulation are called graded potentials. Action potentials occur when threshold is reached, causing a depolarization that spreads along the axon, resulting in synaptic activity at the axon terminal. **33.** Temporal summation is the addition of stimuli that arrive at a single synapse in rapid succession. Spatial summation occurs when simultaneous stimuli at multiple synapses have a cumulative effect on membrane potential.

CHAPTER 12

Section Reviews

Section 1 Review

1. white matter; **2.** dorsal root ganglion; **3.** lateral white column; **4.** posterior gray horn; **5.** lateral gray horn; **6.** anterior gray horn; **7.** posterior median sulcus; **8.** central canal; **9.** sensory nuclei;

ANSWERS

10. motor nuclei; **11.** anterior gray commissure; **12.** ventral root; **13.** anterior white commissure; **14.** anterior median fissure; **15.** anterior view; **16.** radial nerve; **17.** ulnar nerve; **18.** median nerve; **19.** posterior view; **20.** columns; **21.** conus medullaris; **22.** nerves; **23.** meninges; **24.** cauda equina; **25.** brachial plexus; **26.** dura mater; **27.** perineurium; **28.** gray ramus

Section 2 Review

1. divergence; **2.** convergence; **3.** serial processing; **4.** parallel processing; **5.** reverberation; **6.** receptor; **7.** sensory neuron; **8.** interneuron; **9.** spinal cord (CNS); **10.** motor neuron; **11.** effector; **12.** ipsilateral reflex; **13.** withdrawal reflexes; **14.** gamma motor neuron; **15.** flexor reflex; **16.** visceral reflexes; **17.** acquired reflexes; **18.** contralateral reflex; **19.** reciprocal inhibition; **20.** reinforcement; **21.** The withdrawal reflex illustrated in the reflex arc illustration is an innate, somatic, polysynaptic, spinal reflex.

Chapter Review Questions

1. gray matter; **2.** white matter; **3.** ventral root; **4.** spinal nerve; **5.** dorsal root ganglion; **6.** dorsal root; **7.** sympathetic ganglion; **8.** dorsal ramus; **9.** pia mater; **10.** arachnoid; **11.** dura mater; **12.** true; **13.** false; **14.** false; **15.** true; **16.** false; **17.** c; **18.** c; **19.** b; **20.** d; **21.** d; **22.** a; **23.** b; **24.** b; **25.** b; **26.** a; **27.** Shingles is caused by the varicella-zoster virus (VZV), the same virus that causes chickenpox. Symptoms include a painful rash and blisters whose distribution corresponds to the affected sensory nerve and its associated dermatome. **28.** The student bumped her ulnar nerve as it passed behind the medial epicondyle of the humerus. She is experiencing pain in the fourth and fifth finger, as well as the medial hand. **29.** Spinal nerve C_1 exits superior to vertebra C_1. Spinal nerve C_8 exits inferior to vertebra C_7. Therefore, there are eight cervical nerves but only seven cervical vertebrae.

30. Cerebrospinal fluid is located in the subarachnoid space. It functions as a shock absorber and a diffusion medium for dissolved gases, nutrients, chemical messengers, and wastes.

CHAPTER 13

Section Reviews

Section 1 Review

1. precentral gyrus; **2.** frontal lobe; **3.** lateral sulcus; **4.** temporal lobe; **5.** pons; **6.** central sulcus; **7.** postcentral gyrus; **8.** parietal lobe; **9.** occipital lobe; **10.** cerebellum; **11.** medulla oblongata; **12.** olfactory bulb (associated with cranial nerve I, olfactory), S; **13.** oculomotor (III), M; **14.** trigeminal (V), B; **15.** facial (VII), B; **16.** glossopharyngeal (IX), B; **17.** vagus (X), B; **18.** optic (II), S; **19.** trochlear (IV), M; **20.** abducens (VI), M; **21.** vestibulocochlear (VIII), S; **22.** hypoglossal (XII), M; **23.** accessory (XI), M; **24.** thalamus; **25.** arcuate fibers; **26.** fornix; **27.** commissural fibers; **28.** basal nuclei; **29.** The sensory innervation of the nasal lining, or nasal mucosa, is by way of the maxillary branch of the trigeminal nerve (V). Irritation of the nasal lining increases the frequency of action potentials along the maxillary branch of the trigeminal nerve through the semilunar ganglion to reach centers in the midbrain, which in turn excite the neurons of the reticular activating system (RAS). Increased activity by the RAS can raise the cerebrum back to consciousness.

Section 2 Review

1. free nerve ending; **2.** root hair plexus; **3.** tactile discs; **4.** tactile corpuscle; **5.** Ruffini corpuscle; **6.** lamellated corpuscle; **7.** anterior; **8.** posterior; **9.** lateral corticospinal tract of corticospinal pathway (conscious control of skeletal muscles throughout the body); **10.** rubrospinal tract of lateral pathway (subconscious regulation of muscle tone and movement of distal limb muscles); **11.** reticulospinal tract of medial pathway (subconscious regulation of muscle tone, and movements of the neck, trunk, and proximal limb muscles); **12.** vestibulospinal tract of medial pathway (subconscious regulation of muscle tone, and movements of the neck, trunk, and proximal limb muscles); **13.** tectospinal tract of medial pathway (subconscious regulation of muscle tone, and movements of the neck, trunk, and proximal limb muscles in response to bright lights, sudden movements, and loud noises); **14.** anterior corticospinal tract of corticospinal pathway (conscious control of skeletal muscles throughout the body); **15.** posterior column pathway (carries sensations of fine touch, pressure, vibration, and proprioception); **16.** posterior spinocerebellar tract of spinocerebellar pathway (carries proprioceptive information about the position of skeletal muscles, tendons, and joints); **17.** lateral spinothalamic tract of spinothalamic pathway (carries pain and temperature sensations); **18.** anterior spinocerebellar tract of spinocerebellar pathway (carries proprioceptive information about the position of skeletal muscles, tendons, and joints); **19.** anterior spinothalamic tract of spinothalamic pathway (carries crude touch and pressure sensations); **20.** Injuries to the primary motor cortex eliminate the ability to exert fine control over motor units, but gross movements may still be produced by cerebral nuclei using the reticulospinal or rubrospinal tracts.

Chapter Review Questions

1. frontal lobe; **2.** corpus callosum; **3.** thalamus; **4.** hypothalamus; **5.** optic chiasm; **6.** mammillary body; **7.** midbrain; **8.** pons; **9.** precentral gyrus; **10.** central sulcus; **11.** postcentral gyrus; **12.** parietal lobe; **13.** parieto-occipital sulcus;

14. occipital lobe; **15.** pineal gland; **16.** cerebral aqueduct; **17.** fourth ventricle; **18.** medulla oblongata; **19.** false; **20.** true; **21.** false; **22.** false; **23.** true; **24.** b; **25.** b; **26.** a; **27.** d; **28.** b; **29.** a; **30.** b; **31.** d; **32.** In any inflamed tissue, swelling occurs in the area of the inflammation. The accumulation of fluid in the subarachnoid space can cause damage by pressing against neurons. If the intracranial pressure is excessive, brain damage can occur, and if the pressure involves vital autonomic reflex areas, death could occur. **33.** The nerve that is blocked when a dentist works on a tooth in the bottom jaw would be the mandibular branch of the trigeminal nerve (V). This is a mixed nerve. Other sensory areas that could be affected by the injection are the inferior gums, lips, and portions of the tongue and palate. Motor functions that could be affected are the muscles of mastication.

CHAPTER 14

Section Reviews

Section 1 Review

1. cervical sympathetic ganglia; **2.** sympathetic chain ganglia; **3.** coccygeal ganglia; **4.** cardiopulmonary splanchnic nerves; **5.** cardiac and pulmonary plexuses; **6.** celiac ganglion; **7.** superior mesenteric ganglion; **8.** splanchnic nerves; **9.** inferior mesenteric ganglion; **10.** sympathetic division; **11.** thoracolumbar division; **12.** thoracic nerves; **13.** lumbar nerves; **14.** parasympathetic division; **15.** craniosacral division; **16.** cranial nerves III, VII, IX, X; **17.** sacral nerves; **18.** enteric nervous system; **19.** f; **20.** g; **21.** h; **22.** b; **23.** a; **24.** c; **25.** e; **26.** d

Section 2 Review

1. limbic system and thalamus; **2.** hypothalamus; **3.** pons; **4.** spinal cord T_1–L_2; **5.** complex visceral reflexes; **6.** vasomotor; **7.** coughing; **8.** respiratory;

9. sympathetic visceral reflexes; 10. parasympathetic visceral reflexes; 11. P; 12. P; 13. S; 14. P; 15. S; 16. S; 17. P; 18. S; 19. S; 20. S; 21. P; 22. S; 23. P; 24. Even though most sympathetic postganglionic fibers are adrenergic, releasing norepinephrine, a few are cholinergic, releasing acetylcholine. This distribution of the cholinergic fibers by the sympathetic division provides a method of regulating sweat gland secretion and selectively controlling blood flow to skeletal muscles while reducing the flow to other tissues in a body wall to maintain homeostasis.

Chapter Review Questions

1. preganglionic neurons; 2. preganglionic fibers; 3. sympathetic ganglion; 4. ganglionic neurons; 5. postganglionic fibers; 6. parasympathetic ganglion; 7. acetylcholine; 8. norepinephrine; 9. epinephrine; 10. false; 11. true; 12. false; 13. false; 14. false; 15. true; 16. c; 17. d; 18. a; 19. c; 20. a; 21. c; 22. b; 23. a; 24. b; 25. c; 26. a; 27. a; 28. Visceral reflex arcs include a receptor, a sensory neuron, a processing center of one or more interneurons, and two or more visceral motor neurons. Short reflexes bypass the CNS entirely, and control very simple motor responses in one small part of a target organ. Long reflexes deliver information to the CNS along the dorsal roots of spinal nerves, within the sensory branches of cranial nerves, and within the autonomic nerves that innervate visceral effectors. Long reflexes predominate and are responsible for coordinating responses involving multiple organ systems. 29. There are many differences between the somatic and autonomic nervous systems. Three of the differences are the following: the somatic nervous system exerts control only over skeletal muscle, while the autonomic nervous system controls smooth muscle, glands, cardiac muscle, and adipocytes; somatic nervous system effector activity involves an upper motor neuron in the CNS and a lower motor neuron in the PNS, while autonomic nervous system effector activity involves an upper motor neuron in the CNS, and two lower motor neurons in the PNS; and the somatic nervous system uses only ACh at its target organ, while the autonomic nervous system uses ACh, epinephrine, and norepinephrine. 30. The cranial nerves associated with the parasympathetic division are cranial nerves III, VII, IX, and X. The sacral nerves associated with the parasympathetic division are S_2, S_3, and S_4.

CHAPTER 15

Section Reviews

Section 1 Review
1. umami; 2. sour; 3. bitter; 4. salty; 5. sweet; 6. vallate papillae; 7. foliate papillae; 8. fungiform papillae; 9. filiform papillae; 10. e; 11. i; 12. f; 13. m; 14. a; 15. c; 16. k; 17. j; 18. l; 19. h; 20. g; 21. b; 22. d; 23. The olfactory sensory receptor cells are specialized neurons whose cilia-shaped dendrites contain receptor proteins. The binding of odorant molecules to the receptor proteins results in a depolarization of the receptor cell and the production of action potentials. In contrast, the membranes of the sensory receptor cells for taste, vision, equilibrium, and hearing are inexcitable and do not generate action potentials. These cells all form synapses with the processes of sensory neurons, which depolarize and produce action potentials when stimulated by chemical transmitters (neurotransmitters).

Section 2 Review
1. external ear; 2. middle ear; 3. internal ear; 4. auricle; 5. external acoustic meatus; 6. elastic cartilage; 7. tympanic membrane; 8. auditory ossicles (malleus, incus, and stapes); 9. tympanic cavity; 10. petrous part of temporal bone; 11. vestibulocochlear nerve (VIII); 12. cochlea; 13. auditory tube; 14. scala vestibuli; 15. vestibular membrane; 16. cochlear duct; 17. organ of Corti; 18. basilar membrane; 19. scala tympani; 20. spiral ganglion; 21. The rapid descent in the elevator causes the otoliths in the macula of the saccule of each vestibule to slide upward, producing the sensation of downward vertical motion. When the elevator abruptly stops, the otoliths do not. It takes a few seconds for them to come to rest in the normal position. As long as the otoliths are displaced, you will perceive movement.

Section 3 Review
1. posterior cavity; 2. choroid; 3. fovea; 4. optic nerve; 5. optic disc; 6. retina; 7. sclera; 8. fornix; 9. palpebral conjunctiva; 10. ocular conjunctiva; 11. ciliary body; 12. iris; 13. lens; 14. cornea; 15. ciliary zonule (suspensory ligaments); 16. ora serrata; 17. l; 18. k; 19. g; 20. h; 21. o; 22. i; 23. f; 24. d; 25. n; 26. m; 27. j; 28. b; 29. a; 30. c; 31. e; 32. Light falling on the eye passes through the cornea and strikes the photoreceptors of the retina, bleaching (breaking down) many molecules of the pigment rhodopsin into retinal and opsin. After an intense exposure to light, a photoreceptor cannot respond to further stimulation until its rhodopsin molecules have been regenerated by the conversion of retinal molecules to their original shape and recombination with opsin molecules. The "ghost" image remains until the rhodopsin molecules are regenerated.

Chapter Review Questions

1. pigmented part of the retina; 2. central retinal artery; 3. optic nerve; 4. central retinal vein; 5. neural part of the retina; 6. optic disc (blind spot); 7. ganglion cell; 8. sclera; 9. choroid; 10. false; 11. false; 12. true; 13. false; 14. true; 15. true; 16. c; 17. b; 18. a; 19. c; 20. b; 21. The four primary taste sensations are salt, sweet, sour, and bitter. The two other taste sensations that have been identified are umami and water. 22. A cataract is a condition in which the lens loses its transparency. This can be caused by injury, radiation, or a reaction to drugs. Senile cataracts are a natural consequence of aging and are the most common form. Cataracts may be treated with surgery, which involves removing the lens and then replacing it with an artificial substitute. Vision is then refined with glasses or contact lenses. 23. Otitis media is a middle ear infection caused by microorganisms traveling along the auditory tube from the nasopharynx to the middle ear.

CHAPTER 16

Section Reviews

Section 1 Review
1. catecholamines; 2. thyroid hormones; 3. tryptophan derivatives; 4. peptide hormones; 5. short polypeptides; 6. glycoproteins; 7. small proteins; 8. lipid derivatives; 9. eicosanoids; 10. steroid hormones; 11. transport proteins; 12. c; 13. e; 14. f; 15. g; 16. j; 17. h; 18. b; 19. i; 20. a; 21. d; 22. thymus; 23. pineal gland; 24. pancreatic islet; 25. hypothalamus; 26. kidney; 27. adrenal gland; 28. pituitary gland; 29. gonad

Section 2 Review
1. release of natriuretic peptides; 2. suppression of thirst; 3. Na^+ and H_2O loss from kidneys; 4. decreased blood pressure; 5. increased fluid loss; 6. decreasing blood pressure and volume; 7. erythropoietin released; 8. renin released; 9. increased red blood cell production; 10. aldosterone secreted; 11. ADH secreted; 12. increasing blood pressure and volume; 13. c; 14. g; 15. a; 16. e;

17. j; **18.** d; **19.** i; **20.** b; **21.** f; **22.** h; **23.** (1) The two hormones may have opposing or antagonistic effects, such as occurs between insulin (decreases blood glucose levels) and glucagon (increases blood glucose levels). (2) The two hormones may have an additive or synergistic effect, in which the net result is greater than the sum of each acting alone. An example is the enhanced glucose-sparing action of GH in the presence of glucocorticoids. (3) One hormone may have a permissive effect on another, in which the first hormone is needed for the second hormone to produce its effect. For example, epinephrine cannot alter the rate of tissue energy consumption without the presence of thyroid hormones. (4) The hormones may have integrative effects, in which the hormones may produce different but complementary results in specific tissues and organs. An example is the differing effects of calcitriol and parathyroid hormone (PTH) on tissues involved in calcium metabolism; calcitriol increases calcium ion absorption by the intestinal tract, and PTH inhibits osteoblast activity and enhances calcium ion reabsorption by the kidneys.

Chapter Review Questions

1. true; **2.** false; **3.** true; **4.** false; **5.** false; **6.** corticotropin-releasing hormone (CRH); **7.** thyrotropin-releasing hormone (TRH); **8.** growth hormone–releasing hormone (GH–RH); **9.** growth hormone–inhibiting hormone (GH–IH); **10.** prolactin-releasing factor (PRF); **11.** prolactin-inhibiting hormone (PIH); **12.** gonadotropin-releasing hormone (GnRH); **13.** adrenocorticotropic hormone (ACTH); **14.** glucocorticoids (steroid hormones); **15.** thyroid-stimulating hormone (TSH); **16.** thyroid hormones; **17.** growth hormone (GH); **18.** somatomedins; **19.** prolactin (PRL); **20.** follicle-stimulating hormone (FSH); **21.** luteinizing hormone (LH); **22.** inhibin;

23. testosterone; **24.** estrogen; **25.** progesterone; **26.** inhibin; **27.** melanocyte-stimulating hormone; **28.** oxytocin (OXT); **29.** antidiuretic hormone (ADH); **30.** b; **31.** d; **32.** d; **33.** a; **34.** b; **35.** d; **36.** The kidney releases hormones that function to regulate red blood cell production and the rate of calcium and phosphate absorption by the intestinal tract. **37.** Calcitonin decreases blood calcium levels. Parathyroid hormone increases blood calcium levels.

CHAPTER 17

Section Reviews

Section 1 Review
1. f; **2.** l; **3.** j; **4.** o; **5.** b; **6.** g; **7.** a; **8.** i; **9.** k; **10.** m; **11.** n; **12.** c; **13.** e; **14.** h; **15.** d

Section 2 Review
1. plasma; **2.** water; **3.** solutes; **4.** proteins; **5.** electrolytes, glucose, urea; **6.** albumins; **7.** globulins; **8.** fibrinogen; **9.** formed elements; **10.** erythrocytes; **11.** leukocytes; **12.** platelets; **13.** neutrophils; **14.** basophils; **15.** monocytes; **16.** eosinophils; **17.** lymphocytes; **18.** e; **19.** f; **20.** a; **21.** k; **22.** b; **23.** j; **24.** l; **25.** c; **26.** d; **27.** g; **28.** i; **29.** h; **30.** During differentiation, the red blood cells of humans (and other mammals) lose most of their organelles, including nuclei and ribosomes. As a result, mature circulating RBCs can neither divide nor synthesize the structural proteins and enzymes required for cellular repairs.

Chapter Review Questions

1. monocyte; **2.** neutrophil; **3.** erythrocyte, or red blood cell; **4.** lymphocyte; **5.** basophil; **6.** eosinophil; **7.** false; **8.** false; **9.** true; **10.** false; **11.** true; **12.** a; **13.** c; **14.** a; **15.** d; **16.** b; **17.** b; **18.** b; **19.** The two types of leukemias are characterized by elevated levels of circulating WBCs. Myeloid leukemia is

characterized by the presence of abnormal granulocytes (neutrophils, eosinophils, and basophils) or other cells of the bone marrow. Lymphoid leukemia involves lymphocytes and their stem cells. **20.** Blood stabilizes and maintains body temperature by absorbing and redistributing the heat produced by active skeletal muscles. If body temperature is high, the heat will be lost across the surface of the skin. If body temperature is low, the warm blood is directed to the brain and to other temperature-sensitive organs. **21.** Type A blood has surface antigen A and anti-B plasma antibody; type B blood has surface antigen B and anti-A plasma antibody; type AB blood has both A and B surface antigens and neither anti-A nor anti-B plasma antibodies; and type O blood is lacking A and B surface antigens, and has both anti-A and anti-B plasma antibodies.

CHAPTER 18

Section Reviews

Section 1 Review
1. artery; **2.** vein; **3.** smooth muscle; **4.** internal elastic membrane; **5.** endothelium; **6.** tunica intima; **7.** tunica media; **8.** tunica externa, or tunica adventitia; **9.** e; **10.** i; **11.** j; **12.** g; **13.** a; **14.** k; **15.** b; **16.** h; **17.** l; **18.** c; **19.** d; **20.** f; **21.** Contraction or relaxation of the smooth muscle cells in precapillary sphincters control the blood flow into capillaries. During exercise, certain precapillary sphincters will relax to allow more blood flow into the working muscles to meet their metabolic needs, and into the skin to help with cooling. Other precapillary sphincters will contract to decrease blood flow into nonessential organs such as the digestive viscera. In cold temperatures, precapillary sphincters in the periphery and skin will contract to decrease blood flow to these areas and conserve heat.

Section 2 Review
1. common carotid; **2.** subclavian; **3.** brachiocephalic trunk; **4.** brachial; **5.** radial; **6.** popliteal; **7.** fibular (peroneal); **8.** aortic arch; **9.** celiac trunk; **10.** renal; **11.** common iliac; **12.** external iliac; **13.** femoral; **14.** anterior tibial **15.** vertebral; **16.** internal jugular; **17.** brachiocephalic; **18.** axillary; **19.** cephalic; **20.** median antebrachial; **21.** ulnar; **22.** great saphenous; **23.** fibular (peroneal); **24.** superior vena cava; **25.** inferior vena cava; **26.** internal iliac; **27.** deep femoral; **28.** posterior tibial

Chapter Review Questions

1. internal carotid artery; **2.** basilar artery; **3.** vertebral artery; **4.** anterior communicating artery; **5.** anterior cerebral artery; **6.** posterior communicating artery; **7.** posterior cerebral artery; **8.** cerebral arterial circle, or circle of Willis; **9.** d; **10.** b; **11.** d; **12.** c; **13.** a; **14.** d; **15.** a; **16.** b; **17.** A brachiocephalic artery is not needed on the left side of the aortic arch because the majority of the heart lies to the left of midline; this allows the left common carotid artery and left subclavian artery to have direct access to the head and left upper limb, respectively. **18.** Blood volume is distributed throughout the body as follows: 64 percent in the systemic venous system, 9 percent in the pulmonary circuit, 7 percent in the heart, 13 percent in the systemic arterial circuit, and 7 percent in systemic capillaries. **19.** The hepatic portal system directs blood with absorbed nutrients from the digestive system to the liver for processing.

CHAPTER 19

Section Reviews

Section 1 Review
1. aortic arch; **2.** superior vena cava; **3.** right pulmonary arteries; **4.** ascending aorta; **5.** fossa ovalis; **6.** opening of coronary sinus; **7.** right atrium; **8.** pectinate

muscles; **9.** tricuspid valve cusp; **10.** chordae tendineae; **11.** papillary muscle; **12.** right ventricle; **13.** inferior vena cava; **14.** pulmonary trunk; **15.** pulmonary valve; **16.** left pulmonary arteries; **17.** left pulmonary veins; **18.** left atrium; **19.** aortic valve; **20.** bicuspid valve cusp; **21.** left ventricle; **22.** interventricular septum; **23.** trabeculae carneae; **24.** moderator band; **25.** g; **26.** h; **27.** j; **28.** a; **29.** d; **30.** i; **31.** b; **32.** c; **33.** f; **34.** e; **35.** (a) deoxygenated blood flow: right atrium → right atrioventricular valve (tricuspid valve) → right ventricle → pulmonary semilunar valve. (b) oxygenated blood flow: left atrium → left atrioventricular valve (bicuspid valve) → left ventricle → aortic semilunar valve.

Section 2 Review

1. d; **2.** c; **3.** a; **4.** g; **5.** b; **6.** j; **7.** i; **8.** f; **9.** e; **10.** h; **11.** left AV valve closes; **12.** increasing; **13.** decreasing; **14.** less than; **15.** aortic valve is forced open; **16.** aorta; **17.** ventricular systole

Section 3 Review

1. f; **2.** i; **3.** b; **4.** a; **5.** c; **6.** e; **7.** l; **8.** g; **9.** k; **10.** h; **11.** d; **12.** j; **13.** d; **14.** a; **15.** j; **16.** h; **17.** b; **18.** e; **19.** i; **20.** c; **21.** f; **22.** g

Chapter Review Questions

1. true; **2.** false; **3.** false; **4.** true; **5.** true; **6.** c; **7.** a; **8.** b; **9.** c; **10.** d; **11.** b; **12.** a; **13.** b; **14.** a; **15.** d; **16.** The regurgitation of blood into the atria as the ventricles contract is prevented as the papillary muscles contract and pull on the chordae tendineae. **17.** SA node → internodal pathways → AV node → AV bundle → right and left bundle branches → Purkinje fibers; **18.** The epicardium, or visceral pericardium, is a mesothelial serous membrane that covers the outer surface of the heart. The myocardium is the middle layer of the heart and contains cardiac muscle tissue, blood vessels, and nerves. The endocardium is made of simple squamous epithelium (endothelium) and lines the inner surface of the heart.

19. Sympathetic stimulation increases heart rate and force of contraction (contractility). Parasympathetic stimulation decreases heart rate and force of contraction. **20.** The first heart sound is "lubb" (S$_1$) and marks the start of ventricular contraction. The AV valves closing produce this sound. The second sound is "dupp" (S$_2$) and marks the start of ventricular diastole. This sound is produced by the semilunar valves closing. The third heart sound (S$_3$) is associated with blood flow into the atria. The fourth heart sound (S$_4$) is associated with atrial contraction.

CHAPTER 20

Section Reviews

Section 1 Review

1. tonsil; **2.** cervical lymph nodes; **3.** right lymphatic duct; **4.** thymus; **5.** cisterna chyli; **6.** lumbar lymph nodes; **7.** appendix; **8.** lymphatics of lower limb; **9.** lymphatics of upper limb; **10.** axillary lymph nodes; **11.** thoracic duct; **12.** lymphatics of mammary gland; **13.** spleen; **14.** mucosa-associated lymphoid tissue (MALT); **15.** pelvic lymph nodes; **16.** inguinal lymph nodes; **17.** red bone marrow; **18.** c; **19.** h; **20.** l; **21.** i; **22.** m; **23.** j; **24.** b; **25.** e; **26.** g; **27.** d; **28.** f; **29.** a; **30.** k

Section 2 Review

1. physical barriers; **2.** phagocytes; **3.** immune surveillance; **4.** interferons; **5.** complement system; **6.** inflammation; **7.** fever; **8.** d; **9.** d; **10.** c; **11.** d; **12.** a; **13.** a; **14.** The high body temperatures of a fever may inhibit some viruses and bacteria, or increase their reproductive rate so that the disease runs its course more quickly. High body temperatures also accelerate the body's metabolic processes, which may help to mobilize tissue defenses and speed the repair process.

Section 3 Review

1. c; **2.** k; **3.** l; **4.** i; **5.** b; **6.** a; **7.** g; **8.** m; **9.** d; **10.** f; **11.** e; **12.** h; **13.** j;

14. b; **15.** f; **16.** g; **17.** e; **18.** c; **19.** d; **20.** a; **21.** h; **22.** i

Chapter Review Questions

1. antigen binding site; **2.** variable segment of light chain; **3.** constant segments of light and heavy chains; **4.** heavy chain; **5.** light chain; **6.** disulfide bond; **7.** false; **8.** false; **9.** true; **10.** false; **11.** false; **12.** true; **13.** a; **14.** b; **15.** c; **16.** a; **17.** c; **18.** d; **19.** a; **20.** b; **21.** In graft rejection, T cells are activated by contact with MHC proteins on plasma membranes in the donated tissues. The cytotoxic T cells that develop then attack and destroy the foreign cells. **22.** A cytotoxic T cell (T$_C$ cell) destroys its target cell by first encountering its target antigen bound to a Class I MHC protein. It then attacks it by any one of the following mechanisms: (1) destroying the target cell's membrane through the release of perforins; (2) activating apoptosis in the target cell; (3) disrupting the target cell's metabolism through the release of lymphotoxin. **23.** Multiple injections of certain vaccines are timed to produce primary and then secondary responses of the immune system. In the primary response to the vaccine injection, B cells produce daughter cells that differentiate into plasma cells and memory B cells. The plasma cells produce antibodies, which represent the primary response, but the primary response does not maintain elevated antibody levels for long periods. Subsequent vaccine injections are necessary to trigger secondary responses, when memory B cells differentiate into plasma cells that produce antibody concentrations that remain high much longer.

CHAPTER 21

Section Reviews

Section 1 Review

1. nasal cavity; **2.** hard palate; **3.** pharynx; **4.** glottis; **5.** trachea;

6. right lung; **7.** external nares; **8.** larynx; **9.** primary bronchus; **10.** secondary bronchus; **11.** tertiary bronchi; **12.** visceral pleura; **13.** pulmonary lobule; **14.** bronchioles; **15.** terminal bronchiole; **16.** alveolus; **17.** h; **18.** j; **19.** g; **20.** d; **21.** e; **22.** n; **23.** a; **24.** l; **25.** c; **26.** k; **27.** m; **28.** i; **29.** b; **30.** f

Section 2 Review

1. n; **2.** i; **3.** f; **4.** g; **5.** h; **6.** c; **7.** d; **8.** e; **9.** b; **10.** l; **11.** m; **12.** k; **13.** j; **14.** a; **15.** inspiratory reserve volume (IRV): the amount of air that can be taken in above the tidal volume; **16.** tidal volume (V$_T$): the amount of air inhaled and exhaled during a single respiratory cycle while resting; **17.** expiratory reserve volume (ERV): the amount of air that can be expelled after a completely normal, quiet respiratory cycle; **18.** minimal volume: the amount of air remaining in the lungs if they were to collapse; **19.** inspiratory capacity: the amount of air that can be drawn into the lungs after completing a quiet respiratory cycle; **20.** total lung capacity: the total volume of the lungs; **21.** vital capacity: the maximum amount of air that can be moved into or out of the lungs in a single respiratory cycle; **22.** residual volume: the amount of air remaining in the lungs after a maximal exhalation; **23.** functional residual capacity (FRC): the amount of air that remains in the lungs after completing a quiet respiratory cycle; **24.** External respiration includes all the processes involved in the exchange of oxygen and carbon dioxide between blood, lungs, and the external environment. Pulmonary ventilation, or breathing, is a process of external respiration that involves the physical movement of air into and out of the lungs. Internal respiration is the absorption of oxygen and the release of carbon dioxide by tissue cells.

Chapter Review Questions

1. 40 mm Hg; **2.** 45 mm Hg; **3.** 100 mm Hg; **4.** 40 mm Hg; **5.** 100 mm Hg; **6.** 40 mm Hg;

7. 95 mm Hg; 8. 40 mm Hg; 9. 40 mm Hg; 10. 45 mm Hg; 11. 40 mm Hg; 12. 45 mm Hg; 13. e; 14. l; 15. c; 16. i; 17. j; 18. b; 19. a; 20. d; 21. k; 22. f; 23. h; 24. g; 25. d; 26. a; 27. b; 28. b; 29. d; 30. c; 31. The regions of the pharynx are (1) the nasopharynx, located between the soft palate and the internal nares; (2) the oropharynx, located between the soft palate and the base of the tongue at the level of the hyoid bone; and (3) the laryngopharynx, which is the portion of the pharynx located between the hyoid bone and entrance to the larynx and esophagus. 32. The three ways that carbon dioxide is transported in blood are (1) as carbonic acid, (2) bound to the protein portion of hemoglobin molecules within the RBC, or (3) dissolved in plasma as CO_2. 33. Breathing through the nasal cavity is more desirable than breathing through the mouth because the nasal cavity cleanses, moistens, and warms inhaled air, whereas the mouth does not. Breathing through the mouth eliminates much of the conditioning of inhaled air and increases heat and water loss at every exhalation.

CHAPTER 22

Section Reviews

Section 1 Review
1. mesenteric artery and vein; 2. mesentery; 3. circular fold; 4. mucosa; 5. submucosa; 6. muscularis externa; 7. serosa; 8. d; 9. e; 10. a; 11. g; 12. b; 13. c; 14. i; 15. m; 16. l; 17. f; 18. n; 19. j; 20. k; 21. h; 22. With a decrease in smooth muscle tone, general motility along the digestive tract decreases, and peristaltic contractions are weaker.

Section 2 Review
1. crown; 2. neck; 3. root; 4. enamel; 5. dentin; 6. pulp cavity; 7. gingiva; 8. gingival sulcus; 9. cementum; 10. periodontal ligament; 11. root

canal; 12. bone of alveolus; 13. material in jejunum; 14. gastrin; 15. GIP; 16. secretin and CCK; 17. VIP; 18. inhibits; 19. acid production; 20. insulin; 21. bile; 22. intestinal capillaries; 23. gallbladder; 24. nutrient utilization by tissues; 25. Both parietal cells and chief cells are secretory cells found in the gastric glands of the wall of the stomach. However, parietal cells secrete intrinsic factor and hydrochloric acid, whereas chief cells secrete pepsinogen, an inactive proenzyme.

Section 3 Review
1. bile ductule; 2. hepatocytes; 3. central vein; 4. interlobular septum; 5. sinusoid; 6. branch of hepatic artery proper; 7. branch of hepatic portal vein; 8. bile duct; 9. portal area (portal triad); 10. g; 11. h; 12. m; 13. j; 14. l; 15. n; 16. b; 17. e; 18. f; 19. a; 20. i; 21. d; 22. k; 23. c; 24. Saliva (1) continuously flushes and cleans oral surfaces, (2) contains buffers that prevent the buildup of acids produced by bacterial action, and (3) contains antibodies (IgA) and lysozyme, which help control the growth of oral bacterial populations. 25. Such a blockage would interfere with the release of secretions into the duodenum by the pancreas, gallbladder, and liver. The pancreas normally secretes about 1 liter of pancreatic juice, a mixture of a variety of digestive enzymes and buffer solution. The blockage of pancreatic juice would lead to pancreatitis, an inflammation of the pancreas. Extensive damage to exocrine cells by the blocked digestive enzymes would lead to autolysis that could destroy the pancreas and result in the person's death. Blockage of bile secretion from the common bile duct could lead to damage of the wall of the gallbladder by the formation of gallstones and to jaundice because bilirubin from the liver would not be excreted in the bile and, instead, would accumulate in body fluids.

Chapter Review Questions

1. gallbladder; 2. fundus; 3. body; 4. neck; 5. cystic duct; 6. common

bile duct; 7. pancreatic duct; 8. round ligament; 9. left and right hepatic ducts; 10. common hepatic duct; 11. hepatic portal vein and hepatic artery proper; 12. true; 13. false; 14. false; 15. true; 16. false; 17. true; 18. a; 19. b; 20. b; 21. a; 22. d; 23. b; 24. The four different types of teeth are incisors, cuspids, bicuspids, and molars. There are 20 deciduous teeth and 32 permanent teeth. 25. The three phases of gastric secretion are the cephalic phase, the gastric phase, and the intestinal phase. The cephalic phase of gastric secretion begins when you see, smell, taste, or think of food. The CNS is preparing the stomach to receive food. The gastric phase is when food arrives in the stomach. It includes distension of the stomach, an increase in pH, and the presence of undigested materials. The intestinal phase is when chyme first enters the small intestine. 26. The hepatic portal system is a venous portal system in which the hepatic portal vein receives blood from capillaries of most of the abdominal viscera and delivers it to the hepatic sinusoids.

CHAPTER 23

Section Reviews

Section 1 Review
1. d; 2. a; 3. e; 4. k; 5. f; 6. j; 7. g; 8. b; 9. c; 10. h; 11. i; 12. c; 13. e; 14. f; 15. m; 16. b; 17. a; 18. j; 19. l; 20. n; 21. g; 22. k; 23. h; 24. d; 25. i; 26. During fasting or starvation, other tissues shift to fatty acid catabolism or amino acid catabolism, to conserve glucose for neural tissue.

Section 2 Review
1. m; 2. n; 3. j; 4. g; 5. a; 6. k; 7. d; 8. l; 9. f; 10. c; 11. i; 12. h; 13. e; 14. b; 15. d; 16. a; 17. d; 18. b; 19. Essential amino acids are necessary in the diet because the body cannot synthesize them. The body can synthesize nonessential amino acids on demand. 20. (1) Proteins are difficult to break apart because of

their complex three-dimensional structure. (2) The energy yield of proteins (4.32 Cal/g) is less than that of lipids (9.46 Cal/g). (3) The byproducts of protein or amino acid catabolism are ammonium ions, a toxin that can damage cells. (4) Proteins form the most important structural and functional components of cells. Excessive protein catabolism would threaten homeostasis at the cellular to system levels of organization. 21. During the absorptive state, the intestinal mucosa is absorbing nutrients from the digested food. In the postabsorptive state, metabolic activity centers on the mobilization of energy reserves and the maintenance of normal blood glucose levels. 22. Liver cells can break down or synthesize most carbohydrates, lipids, and amino acids. The liver has an extensive blood supply and thus can easily monitor and regulate the blood levels of these nutrients. The liver also stores energy in the form of glycogen. 23. It appears that Claudia is suffering from ketoacidosis as a consequence of her anorexia. Because she is literally starving herself, her body is metabolizing large amounts of fatty acids and amino acids to provide energy and in the process is producing large quantities of ketone bodies (normal metabolites from these catabolic processes). One of the ketones formed is acetone, which can be eliminated through the lungs. Acetone has a fruity aroma, so her breath would also smell fruity. The ketones are organic acids and when they accumulate in the blood, they would decrease the blood pH, and when the ketone bodies spill over into the urine, they would decrease the pH in urine. (In severe cases of ketoacidosis, the ketone bodies may lower blood pH below 7.05, which may cause coma, cardiac arrhythmias, and death.)

Section 3 Review
1. j; 2. d; 3. i; 4. f; 5. m; 6. l; 7. h; 8. k; 9. b; 10. a; 11. c; 12. n; 13. e; 14. g; 15. d; 16. b; 17. c; 18. c; 19. a; 20. a; 21. The

amount of energy used or expended at rest is powered by mitochondrial energy production, which requires oxygen. Using the relationship of 4.825 Calories/L of oxygen, a measurement of the oxygen consumed provides an estimate of the energy expenditure. **22.** The heat-gain center functions in preventing hypothermia, or below-normal body temperature, by conserving body heat and increasing the rate of heat production by the body. **23.** Nonshivering thermogenesis increases the metabolic rate of most tissues through the actions of two hormones, epinephrine and thyroid-stimulating hormone (TSH). In the short term, the heat-gain center stimulates the adrenal medullae to release epinephrine by the sympathetic division of the ANS. Epinephrine quickly increases the breakdown of glycogen (glycogenolysis) in the liver and skeletal muscle, and it increases the metabolic rate of most tissues. The long-term increase in metabolism occurs primarily in children as the heat-gain center adjusts the rate of thyrotropin-releasing hormone (TRH) release by the hypothalamus. When body temperature is low, additional TRH is released, which stimulates the release of TSH by the anterior lobe of the pituitary gland. The thyroid gland then increases its rate of thyroid hormone release, and these hormones increase the rate of catabolism throughout the body.

Chapter Review Questions

1. false; **2.** true; **3.** true; **4.** false; **5.** false; **6.** true; **7.** d; **8.** a; **9.** c; **10.** b; **11.** a; **12.** b; **13.** d; **14.** b; **15.** a; **16.** a; **17.** Some of the energy released during catabolism is captured as ATP, and this ATP can be used as the energy source for anabolism. **18.** A cholesterol level above 200 mg/dL is considered elevated. Elevated cholesterol plus a high LDL:HDL ratio can result in atherosclerotic plaques that can cause heart attacks and strokes. **19.** Too much of a vitamin can produce harmful effects in a condition called hypervitaminosis.

This condition most commonly involves one of the fat-soluble vitamins. **20.** A calorie is the energy needed to raise the temperature of 1 g of water 1°C. A kilocalorie is the amount of energy needed to raise the temperature of 1 kilogram of water 1°C. A Calorie is equal to a kilocalorie.

CHAPTER 24

Section Reviews

Section 1 Review

1. urinary bladder; **2.** nephrons; **3.** renal tubules; **4.** glomerulus; **5.** proximal convoluted tubule; **6.** papillary ducts; **7.** renal medulla; **8.** renal sinus; **9.** major calyces; **10.** ureter; **11.** renal sinus: cavity within kidney that contains calyces, pelvis of the ureter, and segmental vessels; **12.** renal pelvis: funnel-shaped expansion of the superior portion of ureter; **13.** hilum: depression on the medial border of kidney, and site of the apex of the renal pelvis and the passage of segmental renal vessels and renal nerves; **14.** renal papilla: tip of the renal pyramid that projects into a minor calyx; **15.** ureter: tube that conducts urine from the renal pelvis to the urinary bladder; **16.** renal cortex: the outer portion of the kidney containing renal lobules, renal columns (extensions between the pyramids), renal corpuscles, and the proximal and distal convoluted tubules; **17.** renal medulla: the inner, darker portion of the kidney that contains the renal pyramids; **18.** renal pyramid: conical mass of the kidney projecting into the medullary region containing part of the secreting tubules and collecting tubules; **19.** minor calyx: subdivision of major calyces into which urine enters from the renal papillae; **20.** major calyx: primary subdivision of renal pelvis formed from the merging of four or five minor calyces; **21.** kidney lobe: portion of kidney consisting of a renal pyramid and its associated cortical tissue; **22.** renal columns: cortical tissue separating renal pyramids;

23. fibrous capsule (outer layer): covering of the kidney's outer surface and lining of the renal sinus

Section 2 Review

1. f; **2.** j; **3.** h; **4.** i; **5.** g; **6.** a; **7.** e; **8.** c; **9.** d; **10.** b; **11.** nephron: functional unit of the kidney that filters and excretes waste materials from the blood and forms urine; **12.** proximal convoluted tubule: reabsorbs water, ions, and all organic nutrients; **13.** distal convoluted tubule: important site of active secretion; **14.** renal corpuscle: expanded chamber that encloses the glomerulus; **15.** nephron loop: portion of the nephron that produces the concentration gradient in the renal medulla; **16.** collecting system: series of tubes that carry tubular fluid away from the nephron; **17.** collecting duct: portion of collecting system that receives fluid from many nephrons and performs variable reabsorption of water and reabsorption or secretion of sodium, potassium, hydrogen, and bicarbonate ions; **18.** papillary duct: delivers urine to the minor calyx; **19.** The presence of plasma proteins and numerous WBCs in Marissa's urine indicates an increased permeability of the filtration membrane. This condition usually results from inflammation of the filtration membrane within the renal corpuscle. If the condition is temporary, it is probably an acute glomerular nephritis usually associated with a bacterial infection (such as streptococcal sore throat). If the condition is long term, resulting in a nonfunctional kidney, it is referred to as chronic glomerular nephritis. The urine volume would be greater than normal because the plasma proteins increase the osmolarity of the filtrate.

Section 3 Review

1. stretch receptors stimulated; **2.** afferent fibers carry information to sacral spinal cord; **3.** parasympathetic preganglionic fibers carry motor commands; **4.** detrusor muscle contraction stimulated; **5.** sensation relayed to thalamus; **6.** sensation of bladder

fullness delivered to cerebral cortex; **7.** person relaxes external urethral sphincter; **8.** internal urethral sphincter relaxes; **9.** e; **10.** f; **11.** b; **12.** j; **13.** d; **14.** k; **15.** c; **16.** g; **17.** a; **18.** h; **19.** i; **20.** Four primary signs and symptoms of urinary disorders are (1) changes in the volume of urine, (2) changes in the appearance of urine, (3) changes in the frequency of urination, and (4) pain. **21.** cystitis/pyelonephritis: Both conditions involve inflammation and infections of the urinary system, but cystitis refers to the urinary bladder, whereas pyelonephritis refers to the kidney. **22.** stress incontinence/overflow incontinence: Both conditions involve an inability to control urination, but stress incontinence involves periodic involuntary leakage, whereas overflow incontinence involves a continual, slow trickle of urine. **23.** polyuria/proteinuria: Both are abnormal urine conditions, but polyuria is the production of excessive amounts of urine, whereas proteinuria refers to the presence of protein in the urine.

Chapter Review Questions

1. efferent arteriole; **2.** juxtamedullary complex; **3.** afferent arteriole; **4.** glomerular capsule; **5.** capsular space; **6.** initial segment of renal tubule; **7.** parietal layer of glomerular capsule; **8.** visceral layer of glomerular capsule; **9.** false; **10.** true; **11.** true; **12.** false; **13.** false; **14.** true; **15.** d; **16.** a; **17.** b; **18.** b; **19.** c; **20.** b; **21.** a; **22.** a; **23.** The processes of urine production are (1) filtration: blood pressure forces water and solutes across the membranes of the glomerular capillaries and into the capsular space; (2) reabsorption: the transport of water and solutes from the tubular fluid, across the tubular epithelium, and into the peritubular fluid; and (3) secretion: the transport of solutes from the peritubular fluid, across the tubular epithelium, and into the tubular fluid. **24.** The primary process involved in glomerular filtration is basically the same as that regulating fluid and solute movement across capillaries throughout the body: the balance between hydrostatic pressure (fluid pressure) and colloid osmotic pressure (pressure due to materials in solution) on either side of the capillary membrane. **25.** The thin descending limb and the thick ascending limb of the loop of the nephron are very close together and the tubular fluid flows in opposite directions. The exchange that occurs between these segments, called countercurrent multiplication, results in a higher osmotic concentration in the peritubular fluid compared to the tubular fluid in the ascending limb. This process is responsible for creating the concentration gradient in the renal medulla that enables the kidney to produce highly concentrated urine.

CHAPTER 25

Section Reviews

Section 1 Review
1. i; **2.** d; **3.** h; **4.** n; **5.** l; **6.** m; **7.** b; **8.** c; **9.** a; **10.** j; **11.** e; **12.** k; **13.** f; **14.** g; **15.** b; **16.** c; **17.** b; **18.** a; **19.** d; **20.** c; **21.** When tissues are burned, cells are destroyed and the contents of their cytoplasm leak into the interstitial fluid and then move into the blood. Since potassium ions are normally found within cells, damage to a large number of cells releases relatively large amounts of potassium ions into the blood. The elevated potassium level would stimulate cells of the adrenal cortex to produce aldosterone. The elevated levels of aldosterone would promote sodium retention and potassium secretion by the kidneys, thereby accounting for the elevated potassium levels in the patients' urine.

Section 2 Review
1. increased P_{CO_2}; **2.** acidosis; **3.** blood pH decrease; **4.** increased; **5.** secreted; **6.** generated; **7.** decreased; **8.** decreased; **9.** increased; **10.** decreased P_{CO_2}; **11.** alkalosis;

12. blood pH increase; **13.** decreased; **14.** generated; **15.** secreted; **16.** increased; **17.** increased; **18.** decreased; **19.** The young boy has metabolic and respiratory acidosis. The metabolic acidosis resulted primarily from the large amounts of lactic acid generated by the boy's muscles as he struggled in the water. (The dissociation of lactic acid releases hydrogen ions and lactate ions.) Sustained hypoventilation during drowning contributed to both tissue hypoxia and respiratory acidosis. Respiratory acidosis developed as the P_{CO_2} increased in the ECF, increasing the production of carbonic acid and its dissociation into H^+ and $HCO3^-$. Prompt emergency treatment is essential; the usual procedure involves some form of artificial or mechanical respiratory assistance (to increase the respiratory rate and decrease the P_{CO_2} in the ECF) coupled with the intravenous infusion of a buffered isotonic solution that would absorb the hydrogen ions in the ECF and increase body fluid pH.

Chapter Review Questions

1. false; **2.** true; **3.** false; **4.** true; **5.** false; **6.** false; **7.** true; **8.** false; **9.** true; **10.** true; **11.** d; **12.** f; **13.** g; **14.** a; **15.** c; **16.** b; **17.** h; **18.** e; **19.** d; **20.** b; **21.** b; **22.** a; **23.** d; **24.** c; **25.** c; **26.** b; **27.** Fluid balance is when water content in the body remains stable over time. Water gains from the digestive tract must balance with water losses through urination, evaporation at the skin and lungs, feces, and varying degrees of secretion from sweat glands. Mineral balance is the balance between ion absorption, which occurs across the lining of the small intestine and colon, and ion excretion, which is done primarily by the kidneys. Acid–base balance is when the production of hydrogen ions is precisely offset by their loss, and when the pH of body fluids remains within normal limits. **28.** The hypertonic saline solution would cause fluid

to move from the ICF to the ECF, further aggravating the patient's dehydration.

CHAPTER 26

Section Reviews

Section 1 Review
1. prostatic urethra; **2.** ductus deferens; **3.** penile urethra; **4.** penis; **5.** epididymis; **6.** testis; **7.** external urethral orifice; **8.** scrotum; **9.** seminal gland; **10.** prostate gland; **11.** ejaculatory duct; **12.** bulbourethral gland; **13.** j; **14.** h; **15.** i; **16.** l; **17.** m; **18.** k; **19.** n; **20.** b; **21.** c; **22.** a; **23.** f; **24.** d; **25.** e; **26.** g; **27.** Normal levels of testosterone (1) promote the functional maturation of spermatozoa, (2) maintain the accessory organs of the male reproductive tract, (3) are responsible for establishing and maintaining male secondary sex characteristics, (4) stimulate bone and muscle growth, and (5) stimulate sexual behaviors and sexual drive (libido).

Section 2 Review
1. infundibulum; **2.** ovary; **3.** uterine tube; **4.** perimetrium; **5.** myometrium; **6.** endometrium; **7.** uterus; **8.** clitoris; **9.** labium minus; **10.** labium majus; **11.** fornix; **12.** cervix; **13.** external os; **14.** vagina; **15.** j; **16.** d; **17.** l; **18.** i; **19.** b; **20.** f; **21.** n; **22.** m; **23.** e; **24.** a; **25.** h; **26.** c; **27.** k; **28.** g; **29.** The endometrial cells have receptors for estrogens and progesterone and respond to these hormones as if the cells were still in the body of the uterus. Under the influence of estrogens, the endometrial cells proliferate at the beginning of the uterine (menstrual) cycle and begin to develop glands and blood vessels, which then further develop under the control of progesterone. This dramatic increase in tissue size exerts pressure on neighboring tissues or in some other way interferes with their function. It is the recurring expansion of tissue in an abnormal location that causes periodic pain.

Chapter Review Questions

1. ampulla; **2.** ductus deferens; **3.** seminal gland; **4.** prostate gland; **5.** corpus spongiosum; **6.** corpus cavernosum; **7.** epididymis; **8.** testis; **9.** external urethral orifice; **10.** bulbourethral gland; **11.** glans penis; **12.** mons pubis; **13.** prepuce; **14.** clitoris; **15.** labium majus; **16.** urethral opening; **17.** labium minus; **18.** hymen; **19.** vaginal entrance; **20.** false; **21.** true; **22.** true; **23.** false; **24.** true; **25.** false; **26.** c; **27.** c; **28.** b; **29.** a; **30.** d; **31.** a; **32.** Oral contraceptives that contain estrogen and progesterone or only progesterone inhibit GnRH release at the hypothalamus and thus FSH and LH release from the anterior lobe of the pituitary gland through negative feedback. Without FSH, primordial follicles do not begin to develop, and levels of estrogen remain low. An LH surge, triggered by the peaking of estrogen, is necessary for ovulation to occur. If the level of estrogen is not allowed to rise above the critical level, the LH surge will not occur, and thus ovulation will not occur, even if a follicle managed to develop to a stage at which it could ovulate. Any mature follicles would ultimately degenerate, and no new follicles would mature to take their place. Although the ovarian cycle is interrupted, the level of hormones is still adequate to regulate a normal menstrual cycle. **33.** After ovulation the tertiary follicle initially collapses, and the remaining granulosa cells proliferate to create the corpus luteum that secretes progesterone. **34.** The sterilization procedure for men is vasectomy; for women it is tubal ligation. After vasectomy, male sexual function is not affected. Spermatozoa continue to develop, but they are not present in semen because the ductus deferens is now blocked. A man continues to experience an erection as he did before. After tubal ligation, a woman still experiences the menstrual cycle, but the spermatozoa are unable to contact the secondary oocyte because the uterine tubes are now blocked.

CHAPTER 27

Section Reviews

Section 1 Review

1. b; **2.** j; **3.** g; **4.** k; **5.** a; **6.** m; **7.** e; **8.** f; **9.** n; **10.** c; **11.** l; **12.** d; **13.** h; **14.** i; **15.** c; **16.** c; **17.** b; **18.** b; **19.** a; **20.** c; **21.** It is very unlikely that the baby's condition is the result of a viral infection contracted during the third trimester. The development of organ systems occurs during the first trimester, and by the end of the second trimester, most organ systems are fully formed. During the third trimester, the fetus undergoes tremendous growth, but very little new organ formation occurs.

Section 2 Review

1. l; **2.** g; **3.** i; **4.** k; **5.** a; **6.** c; **7.** b; **8.** j; **9.** f; **10.** h; **11.** e; **12.** d; **13.** Tongue-rolling

		Maternal alleles	Maternal alleles
		T	t
Paternal alleles	T	TT	Tt
Paternal alleles	t	Tt	tt

Mom = Tt

Dad = Tt

The possible genotypic and phenotypic ratios of offspring are the following:

1 TT = tongue-roller; 1 in 4 = 25%

2 Tt = tongue-rollers; 2 in 4 = 50%

1 tt = non-tongue-roller; 1 in 4 = 25%

The probability that they will have a child unable to roll his/her tongue is 1 in 4 or 25%.

14. Cystic fibrosis

		Maternal alleles	Maternal alleles
		c	c
Paternal alleles	C	Cc	Cc
Paternal alleles	c	cc	cc

Mom = cc

Dad = Cc

The possible genotypic and phenotypic ratios of offspring are the following:

2 Cc = normal carriers; 2 in 4 = 50%

2 cc = cystic fibrosis; 2 in 4 = 50%

The probability that they will have a child who will be a carrier for CF is 2 in 4 or 50%. (A child has to inherit two copies of the faulty allele to be born with CF.)

Chapter Review Questions

1. false; **2.** true; **3.** false; **4.** true; **5.** false; **6.** true; **7.** false; **8.** false; **9.** b; **10.** b; **11.** d; **12.** a; **13.** b; **14.** d; **15.** c; **16.** d; **17.** The five stages of postnatal development are neonatal (1 month), infancy (1 year), childhood (up to 9 years), adolescence (between 9 and 14 years), and maturity (18 years). **18.** Trisomy 21, or Down's syndrome, is when the affected person has a third chromosome on the 21st pair. Affected people exhibit intellectual disability and physical malformations, including a characteristic facial appearance. There is a direct correlation between maternal age and the risk of having a child with trisomy 21. For a maternal age below 25, the incidence of Down's syndrome approaches 1 in 2000 births, or 0.05 percent. For maternal ages 30–34, the odds increase to 1 in 900, and during ages 35–44 they increase to 1 in 46, or more than 2 percent.